The Next Generation
of AIDS Patients:
Service Needs
and Vulnerabilities

The Next Generation of AIDS Patients: Service Needs and Vulnerabilities has been co-published simultaneously as *Home Health Care Services Quarterly*, Volume 19, Numbers 1/2 2001.

The Next Generation of AIDS Patients: Service Needs and Vulnerabilities

George J. Huba, PhD
Editor

Lisa A. Melchior, PhD
A. T. Panter, PhD
Vivian B. Brown, PhD
David A. Cherin, PhD
W. June Simmons, LCSW
Associate Editors

The Next Generation of AIDS Patients: Service Needs and Vulnerabilities has been co-published simultaneously as *Home Health Care Services Quarterly*, Volume 19, Numbers 1/2 2001.

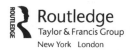

Routledge
Taylor & Francis Group
New York London

The Next Generation of AIDS Patients: Service Needs and Vulnerabilities has been co-published simultaneously as *Home Health Care Services Quarterly*™, Volume 19, Numbers 1/2 2001.

First published by

The Haworth Press, Inc., 10 Alice Street, Binghamton, NY 13904-1580 USA

This edition published 2013 by Routledge

Routledge
Taylor & Francis Group
711 Third Avenue
New York, NY 10017

Routledge
Taylor & Francis Group
2 Park Square, Milton Park
Abingdon, Oxon OX14 4RN

Routledge is an imprint of the Taylor & Francis Group, an informa business

Cover design by Thomas J. Mayshock, Jr.

Library of Congress Cataloging-in-Publication Data

The next generation of AIDS patients : service needs and vulnerabilities / George J. Huba, editor : Lisa A. Melchior, assoc. editor ... [et al.].
     p. cm.
    "Has been co-published simultaneously as Home health care services quarterly, volume 19, numbers 1/2 2001."
    Includes bibliographical references and index.
    ISBN 0-7890-1361-4 (alk. paper)–ISBN 0-7890-1362-2 (alk. paper)
    1. AIDS (Disease)–Patients–Services for–United States. 2. Medically uninsured persons–United States. 3. Poor–Medical care–United States. I. Huba, George J. II. Melchior, Lisa A.
RA643.83 .N49 2001
362.1′969792′00973–dc21
                              2001024048

The Next Generation of AIDS Patients: Service Needs and Vulnerabilities

CONTENTS

Supplemental figures are available online at www.TheMeasurementGroup.com/
HHC/underserved.htm.

Eustache Jean-Louis, MD, MPH
Sandra S. McDonald
Karen Richardson-Nassif, PhD
Geoffrey A. D. Smereck, JD
Anne Stanton, MSW, CSW
Janine Walker, MPH
Katherine Marconi, PhD
A. T. Panter, PhD
David A. Cherin, PhD

Supplemental figures are available online at www.TheMeasurementGroup.com/
HHC/clientsatis.htm.

David A. Cherin, PhD
G. J. Huba, PhD
Judith Steinberg, MD
Peter Reis
Lisa A. Melchior, PhD
Katherine Marconi, PhD
A. T. Panter, PhD

Supplemental figures are available online at www.TheMeasurementGroup.com/
HHC/mcsatis.htm.

ABOUT THE EDITOR

George J. Huba, PhD, is President and Founder of The Measurement Group, a California-based consulting firm that specializes in social policy research, program evaluation, instrument development, and analysis. Dr. Huba was formerly on the faculties of UCLA and the University of Minnesota and Vice President of Research and Development at Western Psychological Services, a test publisher. A licensed psychologist, Dr. Huba received his PhD from Yale University in 1977. He is a Fellow of the Evaluation, Measurement, and Statistics Division and the Addictions Division of the American Psychological Association. Dr. Huba is the author of more than 200 professional works in the technical areas of multivariate statistics, evaluation, the design of computerized expert systems and psychological instrumentation, innovative applications of the Internet for evaluation and information dissemination, and in the content areas of HIV services, substance abuse treatment and prevention, and large-scale human service delivery systems.

ABOUT THE ASSOCIATE EDITORS

Lisa A. Melchior, PhD, is Vice President of The Measurement Group, an applied social research and program evaluation firm. Prior to her work with The Measurement Group, Dr. Melchior coordinated projects in development at Western Psychological Services, a major publisher of psychological and educational tests. A licensed psychologist, Dr. Melchior received her PhD in psychological assessment from the University of Michigan in 1990. She is an active member of the American Psychological Association and the American Public Health Association. Dr. Melchior has published widely in the areas of survey research and evaluation of HIV/AIDS, substance abuse, and mental health services, particularly with respect to services for women and youth and persons with co-occurring disorders.

A. T. Panter, PhD (1989, New York University), is Associate Professor of Psychology in the L. L. Thurstone Psychometric Laboratory at the

University of North Carolina, Chapel Hill. She is also a senior technical consultant at The Measurement Group. Dr. Panter's major research areas are measurement and test theory, multivariate data modeling, evaluation design, and individual differences. She has received several university-wide awards for her innovative approaches to teaching statistics and quantitative methodology to undergraduate and graduate students. Dr. Panter has been extensively involved in The Measurement Group's multi-site evaluation centers and has specialized in work with projects that provide technical assistance and/or health education/training to health care providers. She regularly consults with federal agencies on grant review, is a regular member of NIMH's grant panel on Risk, Prevention, and Health Behavior (RPHB-4), and serves on numerous national committees and editorial boards in the area of social/personality psychology and quantitative methods.

Vivian B. Brown, PhD, is Founder and Chief Executive Officer of PROTOTYPES, Centers for Innovation in Health, Mental Health and Social Services, a multi-facility, multi-service agency with services located throughout California and Washington, DC. Dr. Brown has more than 30 years of experience developing innovative, community-based services including Community Mental Health Centers and crisis intervention centers; residential, day treatment and outpatient drug abuse treatment services; HIV/AIDS outreach, prevention and interventions for women; specialized services for women, their children and their families; mental health treatment and specialized dual diagnosis interventions; and trauma and domestic violence prevention and intervention services. Dr. Brown received her PhD in Clinical Psychology from the University of Southern California. She is Adjunct Associate Professor of Psychiatry at UCLA and a Fellow of the American Psychological Association. She is also a member of numerous federal, state and local advisory committees and was elected Distinguished Practitioner in the National Academy of Practice Psychology.

David A. Cherin, PhD, is Assistant Professor of Social Work at the University of Washington, School of Social Work in Seattle, Washington. He earned his PhD from the University of Southern California and his BA and MSW degrees from California State University, Long Beach. His research focuses on health care delivery and service systems with a focus on chronically ill and terminal patients. He is published in a number of professional journals including *Administration in Social Work,*

Drugs & Society and *Home Health Care Services Quarterly.* He is currently the Principal Investigator of a National Institute of Mental Health grant exploring interventions to reduce and prevent symptom distress that compromise quality of life for terminal patients. He teaches in the areas of policy, organizational practice and research. Prior to receiving his MSW and PhD, Dr. Cherin was a healthcare executive with a major investor-owned hospital chain, American Medical International. Over a 19 year career he was actively engaged in hospital administration, mergers and acquisitions and clinical quality improvement programs.

W. June Simmons, LCSW, is a visionary in developing innovative approaches to health care delivery in the new century as President/CEO of the non-profit Partners in Care Foundation. Throughout her distinguished career, she has been instrumental in creating, funding and operating forward-looking health and social services programs. As head of the Foundation, June Simmons takes an active role in developing initiatives and pro-active programs which meet the mutual needs of patient populations and health care delivery networks to encourage cost-effective, patient-friendly integration of care from hospital to home. Under her leadership, the Foundation has been awarded major grants to investigate and evaluate new models of health care delivery particularly in managed care environments.

In addition, June Simmons currently serves on major national and local technical committees, panels and advisory boards including the Council on Social Work Education Gerontology Project, American Association of Colleges of Nursing/Hartford Institute, L. A. Care Health Plan, Robert Wood Johnson Foundation, California Healthcare Foundation–Managed Care and the Elderly, John A. Hartford Foundation, Community Coalition for Long Term Care, and Hospice of Pasadena, among others. She is also Editor of *Home Health Care Services Quarterly–The Journal of Community Care* and is the author and co-author of many articles published in major scholarly journals as well as a frequent speaker at industry conferences and seminars. She has been recognized for her leadership in innovation and management by academic and national professional organizations.

EDITORIAL

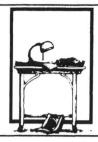

This volume deals with the emerging profile of HIV/AIDS and the needs of this population. It focuses on the needs of AIDS patients who remain vulnerable to both the disease and mainstream treatment regimens and who have been underserved by both traditional models of community-based services and service delivery programs. The face of AIDS and the nature of AIDS treatment and care have changed dramatically over the last half of this decade. New and innovative approaches to care were inevitable as a product of these changes. Medical models of care, effectively utilized in the earlier waves of AIDS, are not effective on their own in reaching women of color or substance abusers. Programs designed to focus on prevention and treatment of AIDS for these populations must wrap services within the psychosocial contexts of today's AIDS patients. This volume is focused therefore on describing the current demographics of AIDS and detailing innovative programs attempting to reach AIDS patients and profiling the agencies and leaders who have created innovative programs of care.

The innovative programs presented herein were funded by the Ryan

[Haworth co-indexing entry note]: "Editorial." Simmons, W. June. Co-published simultaneously in *Home Health Care Services Quarterly* (The Haworth Press, Inc.) Vol. 19, No. 1/2, 2001, pp. xvii-xviii; and: *The Next Generation of AIDS Patients: Service Needs and Vulnerabilities* (ed: George J. Huba et al.) The Haworth Press, Inc., 2001, pp. xvii-xviii. Single or multiple copies of this article are available for a fee from The Haworth Document Delivery Service [1-800-342-9678, 9:00 a.m. - 5:00 p.m. (EST). E-mail address: getinfo@haworthpressinc.com].

White Care Act as demonstration projects under the Special Projects of National Significance. All the projects presented in this volume were part of a five year, cross-cutting evaluation that took the first national look at critical issues of access, risk factors, needs and treatment satisfaction for traditionally underserved individuals with AIDS. The projects described also shared a charge to develop, connect and configure both community-based and acute services in innovative ways. Part of their program mission was to develop methods to reach patients who were underserved by traditional AIDS care and who have historically experienced significant barriers to accessing prevention services and ongoing treatment.

In presenting these projects, we hope to bring attention to the critical need for well-organized, comprehensive and innovative treatment programs in meeting the evolving needs of today's AIDS patients. Programs highlighted in this volume assembled continuums of care around the patients they served and blended psychosocial services with biological services to mold seamless systems of treatment. Whether projects were community-based providers of specialty services or comprehensive managed care providers, each project focused on a client-centered approach to both treatment modalities as well as the context of service delivery. Each site dedicated a large portion of their evaluation efforts toward understanding the specific needs of the populations they served and to understanding and eliminating the barriers to treatment experienced by their patients. The outcomes of this work are presented in this volume.

We thank George J. Huba, PhD, of The Measurement Group for serving as Editor. In addition, this volume is further enhanced by a Foreword prepared by Joseph F. O'Neill, MD, MPH, Associate Administrator, and Steven R. Young, MSPH, Deputy Director of the Office of Epidemiology, both of the U.S. Health Resources and Services Administration, HIV/AIDS Bureau. Everyone involved in the preparation of this collection hopes that the information presented will serve the best interests and concerns of AIDS patients and the community-based providers dedicated to providing services.

W. June Simmons

scribed herein provide a significant contribution to the identification of best practices to increase access to and retention in care for new populations affected by HIV.

Joseph F. O'Neill, MD, MPH
Associate Administrator
HIV/AIDS Bureau, HRSA

Steven R. Young, MSPH
Deputy Director
Office of Science and Epidemiology
HIV/AIDS Bureau, HRSA

Foreword

Since the initial authorization of the Ryan White Comprehensive AIDS Resources Emergency (CARE) Act in 1990, the Health Resources and Services Administration's (HRSA) HIV/AIDS program has served a critical role in developing community-based care services and infrastructure for the delivery of necessary medical and support services for uninsured and underinsured, low-income persons with HIV disease. Although substantial gains have been made over the last decade, there remain serious challenges for the future as the nature, treatment and epidemiology of the disease continues to change. Additionally, the continuum of HIV care developed to date has come under criticism for its comprehensiveness as compared to the treatment of other life-threatening or infectious illnesses. It is thus critical to gather information about program effectiveness and cost based on service delivery data to respond effectively and engage new individuals in the care system, provide the highest quality care, and increase service capacity in underserved communities. Lessons learned have specific applicability for the care of persons living with HIV disease and broader potential beyond HIV. They can inform how populations most vulnerable and underrepresented in health services delivery should receive community-based health care.

Within the CARE Act, the Special Projects of National Significance (SPNS) program provides the opportunity to identify and address the needs of, and improve access and reduce barriers to care for, traditionally underserved and vulnerable populations. This is accomplished through the development and evaluation of innovative service delivery models. Results from 17 recently completed SPNS Cooperative Agreement Projects presented in the following articles address populations

[Haworth co-indexing entry note]: "Foreword." O'Neill, Joseph F., and Steven R. Young. Co-published simultaneously in *Home Health Care Services Quarterly* (The Haworth Press, Inc.) Vol. 19, No. 1/2, 2001, pp. xix-xxi; and: *The Next Generation of AIDS Patients: Service Needs and Vulnerabilities* (ed: George J. Huba et al.) The Haworth Press, Inc., 2001, pp. xix-xxi. Single or multiple copies of this article are available for a fee from The Haworth Document Delivery Service [1-800-342-9678, 9:00 a.m. - 5:00 p.m. (EST). E-mail address: getinfo@haworthpressinc.com].

xix

only marginally represented in previous HIV/AIDS studies and data sets.

Each of the 17 projects contributed to a multi-site data pool and cross-cutting evaluation. Although there were quite different management information systems–ranging from paper client records to multiple, and sometimes incompatible, electronic record systems–these projects illustrate how community-based programs can effectively collaborate in multi-site data collection and program evaluation. The collective data are from a diverse set of HIV providers, ranging from AIDS service organizations to neighborhood health centers to large university medical centers to small community-based organizations. As a group, the projects have highlighted the potential uses of public health and clinical data to further contribute to the identification of best practices for community-based HIV care.

As we search for better ways of prolonging the lives of individuals diagnosed with HIV and preventing new infections and co-morbid conditions, the SPNS models provide valuable information. The articles that follow describe mechanisms to identify, engage, and retain individuals in care who demonstrate a very high level of unmet need. They explore effective outreach to those outside the care system, program development and implementation responsive to client needs and barriers to HIV care, as well as resultant changes in client satisfaction and quality of life. Issues of HIV service delivery are addressed for diverse minority populations, those who are homeless, geographically isolated, chemically dependent, face language barriers or attempt to navigate new managed care systems.

Ryan White CARE Act programs operate in an ever-changing arena. The epidemic is increasingly affecting medically underserved minority populations. There has been pressure to provide access to new and rapidly developing clinical advancements. Other public/private financing systems to manage health care delivery and costs affect CARE Act programs. Based on data from these SPNS Cooperative Agreement Projects, it is evident that comprehensive programs responsive to the particular needs of those most affected by HIV and most disadvantaged because of circumstances of poverty can be developed and evaluated for their effectiveness. Federal investment in and findings from innovative models of community-based HIV care de-

Introduction:
Evaluating HIV/AIDS Treatment Programs for Underserved and Vulnerable Patients, Innovative Methods and Findings

G. J. Huba, PhD

In 1994, the U.S. Department of Health and Human Services (DHHS), Health Resources and Services Administration (HRSA), through its Special Projects of National Significance (SPNS) Program, funded 27 innovative models of HIV care. These projects, known collectively as the SPNS Cooperative Agreement, represented a diverse group of organizations with common goals: to improve access to care, health, and quality of life for traditionally underserved populations living with HIV/AIDS.

Indeed, the Cooperative Agreement Projects reached a high-need population. Enrollees across the various programs had the following characteristics: 72.5% were people of color, 88.9% lacked private insurance, 85.7% were unemployed or unable to work due to a disabil-

G. J. Huba is affiliated with The Measurement Group, Culver City, CA. Address correspondence to: G. J. Huba, PhD, The Measurement Group, 5811A Uplander Way, Culver City, CA 90230 (E-mail: *ghuba@TheMeasurementGroup.com*).

This work was supported in part by the Health Resources and Services Administration (HRSA), HIV/AIDS Bureau (HAB), Special Projects of National Significance (SPNS) Grant No. 5 U90 HA 00030-05. This publication's contents are solely the responsibility of the authors and do not necessarily represent the official view of the funding agency.

[Haworth co-indexing entry note]: "Introduction: Evaluating HIV/AIDS Treatment Programs for Underserved and Vulnerable Patients, Innovative Methods and Findings." Huba, G. J. Co-published simultaneously in *Home Health Care Services Quarterly* (The Haworth Press, Inc.) Vol. 19, No. 1/2, 2001, pp. 1-6; and: *The Next Generation of AIDS Patients: Service Needs and Vulnerabilities* (ed: George J. Huba et al.) The Haworth Press, Inc., 2001, pp. 1-6. Single or multiple copies of this article are available for a fee from The Haworth Document Delivery Service [1-800-342-9678, 9:00 a.m. - 5:00 p.m. (EST). E-mail address: getinfo@haworthpressinc.com].

ity, 54.2% had a history of problem drinking, 44.9% had a history of crack use, 28.2% had a history of heroin use, 56.9% had reported other illicit drug use, 45.3% had less than a high school education, 49.7% had been involved with the criminal justice system, 20.0% had children requiring care, 22.1% had a history of sex work, 42.9% were sex partners of injection drug users, 46.4% were without stable housing, 11.9% had a primary language other than English and 6.0% were under 21 years of age or over 55 years of age. The average score on an index of these service needs-vulnerabilities was 7.13 ($s.d.$ = 2.73, n = 1,060) for males and 6.75 ($s.d.$ = 2.68, n = 1,054) for females (t = 3.23 for the difference, degrees of freedom = 2112, p < .001). Almost all enrollees (87.7%) had four or more need-vulnerability factors (Huba, Melchior, & Panter, 1998-2000).

As part of the cross-cutting evaluation of the projects (see Huba, Melchior, & Panter, 1998-2000; Huba, Melchior, De Veauuse, Hillary, Singer, & Marconi, 1998; Huba, Melchior, Panter, Brown, & Larson, 2000), data have been collected on service needs and perceived barriers to care, service utilization histories, quality of life, program satisfaction, medical history, psychological functioning, and other outcomes from almost 5,000 persons living with HIV/AIDS. Issues described by Huba, Brown, Melchior, Hughes, and Panter (2000) framed the collection of these evaluation data. For this collection we have focused on what types of clients are likely to enter innovative HIV/AIDS programs from the community (the articles on "finding the underserved," "unmet needs," and "barriers to services") and what happens if high-quality, innovative programming is provided (the articles on "service satisfaction"). High-need individuals can be recruited and provided interventions that generate high levels of client-patient satisfaction. Detailed descriptions of the service programs that can produce these results are available on the Internet at *www.TheMeasurementGroup.com/KB.htm* (Huba, Melchior, & Panter, 1998-2000).

This volume highlights pooled data from the efforts of several clusters of projects within this initiative. One such group includes six programs identified as Community-Based Organizations (CBOs). The CBO projects share as a central theme the goal of providing high-quality care for individuals with HIV who belong to groups that are traditionally underserved because of linguistic, cultural, racial, and economic barriers that prevent their full integration into the traditional hospital-based service system. Another group featured here includes three projects that developed specialized medical care models within the context of a continuum of services in a medical clinic. The third group of projects includes four models that focused on providing quality healthcare for persons with HIV/AIDS under capitated systems of reimbursement. This volume also includes an overview of the HRSA HIV/AIDS Bureau (HAB) SPNS Cooperative Agreement grant initiative, and two editorials linking these innovative models of care back to broader issues in providing community-based care for persons with HIV/AIDS.

A growing resource for more information about these innovative HIV care models and their evaluations is available in an online Knowledge Base at *www.TheMeasurementGroup.com/KB.htm*. The Knowledge Base on Innovative Models of HIV/AIDS Care (Huba, Melchior, & Panter, 1998-2000) presents literally thousands of pooled results from the Cooperative Agreement Projects (of which those presented here are but a small subset) and provides a method of rapid and wide information dissemination from this initiative via the Internet. The Knowledge Base builds on many of the results presented in this volume and is continuously updated and expanded. The Knowledge Base not only summarizes data from these projects in a highly accessible format, but also provides links to data collection forms and evaluation methods used to generate the information, as well as links to information about the service models that produced the featured results. I invite you to bookmark this resource and visit it often.

One other item worth noting here is that the predominant analysis methodology used in the articles in this volume is a method called Exhaustive CHAID (Chi-squared Automatic Interaction Detector; Biggs, de Ville, & Suen, 1991). CHAID is a method for analyzing a mixture of continuous data (such as number of service needs) and categorical variables (such as codes for risk behaviors or demographic characteristics). In a very systematic way, CHAID searches data for relationships between the independent and dependent measures. Relationships are determined mechanically in that the sample is split in a way that can be arranged into a decision tree. Homogenous groups of individuals are identified in terms of their levels on the dependent measure. The groups are formed by determining whether they show statistically significant differences on the dependent measure. CHAID is a particularly interesting method for summarizing very complicated data and their interrelationships for audiences which tend to be heterogeneous in their level of methodological training and professional backgrounds because the method yields decision trees which show how the sample can be split into pieces which often have direct clinical interpretations so as to yield different groups of patients with maximally different values on the variable predicted. Thus, the method is useful for generating "types" of individuals likely to have different levels of service need, and types of individuals who have different levels of satisfaction with the programs. And, to the extent that the method cannot generate such types, it means that various grouping factors hoped not to affect one's outcomes from a program (such as gender or sexual orientation or race or specific behaviors) have a minimal impact. It should be recognized that CHAID is a data exploration and *modeling* method and that some decisions are required for its successful use. The data models presented here are supported by literally hundreds of alternate statistical analyses including logistic and multiple linear regressions, general linear models, and log linear modeling analyses presented online at *www.TheMeasurementGroup. com/KB.htm* (Huba, Melchior, & Panter, 1998-2000). Our general technical conclusions about the importance of this model for modeling data from evaluation studies, and the relationship of the generated data models to results from other hypothesis testing statistical methods is summarized in a paper by Huba, Panter, and Melchior (2000) that discusses and illustrates the ability of these modeling methods to "replicate" the results from other traditional technical procedures, as well as discusses key methodological decisions. We conclude that the CHAID models such as those presented here are very useful to summarize a large number of multivariate relationships for heterogeneous audiences of both programmatic and technical professionals.

The work featured in this volume would not be possible without the contributions of a number of key individuals and organizations. First and foremost, funding from the Health Resources and Services Administration in the form of the Cooperative Agreements supported the efforts of the individual service models as well as the Evaluation and Dissemination Center that coordinated the multi-site evaluation (a collaboration of The Measurement Group and PROTOTYPES). Throughout the five years of this initiative, Katherine Marconi, PhD, led the efforts in the Office of Science and Epidemiology within the HRSA HIV/AIDS Bureau, of which Joseph O'Neill, MD, MPH, was Associate Administrator and the head of HRSA's HIV programs. The SPNS

Program itself was overseen initially (1994-1995) by William Grace, PhD, and subsequently by Barney Singer, JD (1996-1998) and Barbara Aranda-Naranjo, PhD (1999-present).

I also thank the Associate Editors for their invaluable work on this volume. Lisa A. Melchior, PhD, of The Measurement Group and A. T. Panter, PhD, of the University of North Carolina Chapel Hill and a Senior Research Consultant to The Measurement Group, worked with me in all phases of the cross-cutting evaluation. Vivian B. Brown, PhD, served multiple roles in the Cooperative Agreement, including that of an Associate Director for the Evaluation and Dissemination Center and Principal Investigator of the PROTOTYPES WomensLink program for women living with HIV/AIDS. David Cherin, PhD, and June Simmons, LCSW, were the Project Director and Principal Investigator, respectively, of the project at the Partners in Care Foundation of Los Angeles. I especially thank June Simmons in her role as Editor of *Home Health Care Services Quarterly* for her assistance in making this volume possible and for working with me on the overall direction for the volume, as well as contributing an article on the usefulness of these results in planning innovative community health services. The associate editors have helped to ensure that the articles included here would be maximally useful and relevant for practitioners and researchers alike. In that respect, I also thank the contribution of the outside reviewers who reviewed these manuscripts and provided helpful comments and suggestions for the authors.

Finally, the production of this volume could not have been accomplished without the hard work of a number of staff at The Measurement Group. I thank Rupinder K. Sidhu, Cindy T. Le, and Kimberly Ishihara for their assistance with manuscript preparation and word processing and Jocelyn Medina and Kate Ellingson for helping me with the primary data modeling analyses. I also wish to note the work of the late Diana E. Brief, PhD, who passed away unexpectedly before the completion of this project. Dr. Brief provided extensive technical assistance to all the projects throughout the course of the Cooperative Agreement so as to maximize the quality of data available to demonstrate the successes of these innovative service models.

REFERENCES

Biggs, D., de Ville, B., & Suen, E. (1991). A method of choosing multiway partitions for classification and decision trees. *Journal of Applied Statistics*, 18, 49-62.

Huba, G. J., Brown, V. B., Melchior, L. A., Hughes, C., & Panter, A. T. (2000). Conceptual issues in implementing and using evaluation in the "real world" setting of a community-based organization for HIV/AIDS services. *Drugs & Society, 16*(1/2), 31-54.

Huba, G. J., Melchior, L. A., & Panter, A. T. (1998-2000). Knowledge Base on HIV/AIDS Care. Online: *www.TheMeasurementGroup.com/KB.htm*.

Huba, G. J., Melchior, L. A., De Veauuse, N., Hillary, K., Singer, B., & Marconi, K. (1998). A national program of AIDS capitated care projects and their evaluation. *Home Health Care Services Quarterly, 17*(1), 3-30.

Huba, G. J., Melchior, L. A., Panter, A. T., Brown, V. B., & Larson, T. L. (2000). A national program of AIDS care projects and their cross-cutting evaluation: The HRSA SPNS Cooperative Agreements. *Drugs & Society, 16*(1/2), 5-29.

Huba, G. J., Panter, A. T., & Melchior, L. A. (2000). Empirical modeling of patient characteristics and services using sample partitioning, interaction detection, or classification tree methods: Practical issues and recommendations. Manuscript in preparation.

Finding the Underserved:
Directions for HIV Care in the Future

Trudy A. Larson, MD
Linda M. Mundy, MD
Lisa A. Melchior, PhD
A. T. Panter, PhD
Vivian B. Brown, PhD
Paul Chase, JD
David A. Cherin, PhD
Tracey Gallagher
Victor F. German, MD, PhD
Eustache Jean-Louis, MD
Jay Kaplan, JD
Sandra S. McDonald
Karen L. Meredith, MPH
Peter Reis
Karen Richardson-Nassif, PhD
Catherine Rohweder, MPH
Geoffrey A. D. Smereck, JD
Anne Stanton, MSW, CSW
Judith Steinberg, MD
Katherine Marconi, PhD
G. J. Huba, PhD

Address correspondence to: G. J. Huba, The Measurement Group, 5811A Uplander Way, Culver City, CA 90230 (E-mail: *ghuba@TheMeasurementGroup.com*).

[Haworth co-indexing entry note]: "Finding the Underserved: Directions for HIV Care in the Future." Larson, Trudy A. et al. Co-published simultaneously in *Home Health Care Services Quarterly* (The Haworth Press, Inc.) Vol. 19, No. 1/2, 2001, pp. 7-27; and: *The Next Generation of AIDS Patients: Service Needs and Vulnerabilities* (ed: George J. Huba et al.) The Haworth Press, Inc., 2001, pp. 7-27. Single or multiple copies of this article are available for a fee from The Haworth Document Delivery Service [1-800-342-9678, 9:00 a.m. - 5:00 p.m. (EST). E-mail address: getinfo@haworthpressinc.com].

SUMMARY. The demographic, behavior, and background characteristics of 4,804 participants in 17 national demonstration projects for HIV medical and/or psychosocial support services were coded for an index of "service need" or possible under-representation in the traditional healthcare system. Fifteen items were coded including status as a person of color, lack of private insurance, unemployment/disability, problem drinking, crack cocaine use, heroin use, other illicit drug use, less than 12 years of education, criminal justice system involvement, children requiring care while the patient receives services, sex work, being the sex partner of an injection drug user, unstable housing, primary language not English, and age less than 21 or over 55 years. Most (87.7%) of the program participants had four or more of these factors present. Through CHAID modeling, those groups with the highest levels of service need and vulnerability were identified. These data suggest that these projects, designed to attract and serve individuals potentially underrepresented in the health services system, had in fact achieved that goal. Implications of the changing demographics of the HIV epidemic for the health service delivery system are discussed. *[Article copies available for a fee from The Haworth Document Delivery Service: 1-800-342-9678. E-mail address: <getinfo@haworthpressinc.com> Website: <http://www.HaworthPress. com> © 2001 by The Haworth Press, Inc. All rights reserved.]*

KEYWORDS. HIV/AIDS, underserved, CHAID

Since the first reports of AIDS in 1982, populations impacted by HIV have grown and changed (Centers for Disease Control and Prevention, 1999). As a result, these changing populations have substantially affected the way in which HIV care is delivered and supported. To understand better the emerging populations and their needs, the U.S. Department of Health and Human Services (DHHS) Health Resources and Services Administration (HRSA) HIV/AIDS Bureau (HAB) funded 27 Innovative Models of HIV/AIDS Care through its Special Projects of National Significance (SPNS) Program (Huba, Melchior, De Veauuse, Hillary, Singer, & Marconi, 1998; Huba, Melchior, Panter, Brown, & Larson, 2000). The individual service models varied, but all shared the goals of increasing access and reducing barriers to HIV/AIDS services. The target populations included women, adolescents, ethnically distinct populations, rural populations, and substance abusers. This article describes the success of these projects in enrolling difficult to reach and traditionally underserved HIV/AIDS populations in care.

The information reported summarizes the demographic characteristics of patients in 17 HIV/AIDS service demonstration projects. This unique population has been previously only marginally represented in other large HIV/AIDS databases and studies (e.g., Bozzette et al., 1998). The data highlight common conditions and circumstances that impact the manner in which HIV care is delivered and suggest intensive patient needs (see also Huba, 2000). Projects were designed to test innovative approaches to serve these needs, to measure a variety of outcomes, and to document the circumstances under which services were delivered. Table 1 provides a short summary of each project. More detailed descriptions of each project and its findings are given on the Internet at *www.TheMeasurementGroup.com/KB.htm* (Huba, Melchior, & Panter, 1998-2000) and by Huba, Melchior, Brown, Larson, and Panter (2000).

Each of the 17 projects represented here targeted different underserved populations. Table 2 summarizes in a very broad way the relative project emphases. The check marks in Table 2 indicate the groups that were specifically targeted by the individual HIV/AIDS service models. Although any of the programs may have certainly provided services to members of a given population (e.g., substance abusers), Table 2 shows the projects that actively conducted outreach and other efforts to engage members of that group in a state-of-the-art program for persons living with HIV/AIDS specifically designed to meet the unique needs of that group.

METHOD

Participants

A total of 4,804 people with HIV/AIDS were enrolled in 17 projects located in 11 geographically diverse metropolitan areas. There were 2,225 females and 2,579 males. The criteria for enrollment varied by site, but all required documentation of HIV-positive serostatus by onsite or referral testing. Data were collected between October 1994 and June 1999.

Both the size and the demographic range of this studied population set it apart from other HIV/AIDS studies. Among those individuals who had valid data for each indicator, 72.5% were people of color, 88.9% lacked private insurance, 85.7% were unemployed or unable to

TABLE 1. Synopsis of Projects

Project	Description of Project	Internet Address for More Information
AIDS Healthcare Foundation	AHF has operated four healthcare centers to provide direct medical services to individuals living with HIV/AIDS under a capitated system of care.	*www.TheMeasurementGroup.com/edcpage/ahf.html*
Center for Community Health Education and Research	The CCHER Haitian Community AIDS Outreach Project is a culturally competent psychosocial educational counseling program that has addressed the emotional and educational needs of HIV-positive Haitians in Boston.	*www.TheMeasurementGroup.com/edcpage/ccher.html*
East Boston Neighborhood Health Center	EBNHC has provided coordinated, non-fragmented, comprehensive care to individuals with HIV/AIDS under a capitated system of care.	*www.TheMeasurementGroup.com/edcpage/ebnhc.html*
The Fortune Society	The Fortune Society has delivered culturally and linguistically appropriate services to symptomatic HIV-positive Hispanic prisoners and ex-offenders.	*www.TheMeasurementGroup.com/edcpage/fortune.html*
Indiana Community AIDS Action Network	The ICAAN project helped reduce discriminatory barriers to employment, care, housing, and other social services faced by individuals living with HIV/AIDS.	*www.TheMeasurementGroup.com/edcpage/indiana.html*
Johns Hopkins University School of Medicine	The Johns Hopkins University project reduces financial barriers to adequate care for HIV/AIDS patients without compromising the quality of care.	*www.TheMeasurementGroup.com/edcpage/hopkins.html*
Larkin Street Youth Center	LSYC has reduced barriers to care and has assisted homeless youth in the San Francisco Bay Area in accessing services.	*www.TheMeasurementGroup.com/edcpage/larkin.html*
Michigan Protection and Advocacy Service	The MPAS project trained Community Advocates throughout the state on HIV/AIDS legal issues to improve service delivery systems.	*www.TheMeasurementGroup.com/edcpage/michigan.html*
Outreach, Inc.	Outreach, Inc. has offered a wide array of comprehensive services to African American substance abusers with HIV/AIDS residing in or around housing developments in Atlanta, Georgia.	*www.TheMeasurementGroup.com/edcpage/outreach.html*

Project	Description of Project	Internet Address for More Information
PROTOTYPES	PROTOTYPES WomensLink has reduced barriers and increased access to care for women living with HIV/AIDS through the provision of a comprehensive, "seamless" continuum of care and services.	www.TheMeasurementGroup.com/edcpage/prototypes.html
State University of New York	The project at SUNY Brooklyn has increased counseling and testing of pregnant women and perinatal AZT protocols.	www.TheMeasurementGroup.com/edcpage/suny.html
University of Nevada School of Medicine	The University of Nevada School of Medicine project has prevented or slowed wasting syndrome experienced by individuals living with HIV/AIDS.	www.TheMeasurementGroup.com/edcpage/nevada.html
University of Texas Health Science Center	The University of Texas project has helped positively impact changes in the service delivery systems for families living with, or affected by, HIV/AIDS.	www.TheMeasurementGroup.com/edcpage/texas.html
University of Vermont & State Agricultural College	The University of Vermont & State Agricultural College project has reduced barriers to care experienced by individuals living with HIV in rural areas.	www.TheMeasurementGroup.com/edcpage/vermont.html
Visiting Nurse Association Foundation Los Angeles	VNAF's Transprofessional Model has used an interdisciplinary, case management approach–a blend of curative and palliative services– that has improved services for end-stage AIDS patients.	www.TheMeasurementGroup.com/edcpage/vnf.html
Washington University School of Medicine	The Helena Hatch Special Care Center (HHSCC)–in the Division of Infectious Diseases–is a specialized medical care clinic that has provided coordinated, comprehensive care to adolescent and adult women with HIV/AIDS.	www.TheMeasurementGroup.com/edcpage/washuniv.html
Well-Being Institute	The Well-Being Institute is a comprehensive community-based nursing project reducing access barriers for substance-abusing, HIV-positive women who "fall between the cracks" of the health delivery system in Detroit.	www.TheMeasurementGroup.com/edcpage/wbi.html

11

TABLE 2. HRSA SPNS Cooperative Agreement Projects by Target Populations

	AHF	CCHER	EBNHC	Fortune	ICAAN	Hopkins	LSYC	MPAS	Outreach	PROTO-TYPES	SUNY	UNSOM	UTHSC	UVM	VNAF	HHSCC	WBI
Age Less than 21							✓						✓				
Person of Color	✓	✓	✓	✓	✓	✓	✓	✓	✓	✓	✓	✓	✓	✓	✓	✓	✓
Language Not English		✓	✓	✓						✓			✓				
Children Needing Care	✓	✓								✓	✓		✓			✓	✓
No High School Completion	✓	✓	✓	✓	✓	✓	✓	✓	✓	✓	✓	✓	✓	✓	✓	✓	✓
Unemployed	✓	✓	✓	✓	✓	✓	✓	✓	✓	✓	✓	✓	✓	✓	✓	✓	✓
Public Supported Medical Services	✓	✓	✓	✓	✓	✓	✓	✓	✓	✓	✓	✓	✓	✓	✓	✓	✓
Alcohol Problem	✓	✓	✓	✓		✓	✓		✓	✓			✓				✓
Heroin User		✓	✓	✓		✓	✓		✓	✓			✓				✓
Crack User		✓	✓	✓		✓	✓		✓	✓			✓				✓
Other Illicit Drug Use	✓	✓	✓	✓		✓	✓		✓	✓			✓				✓
Criminal Justice System Involvement				✓					✓	✓							
Sex Worker							✓		✓	✓							✓
Unstable Housing	✓	✓	✓	✓	✓	✓	✓	✓	✓	✓	✓	✓	✓	✓	✓	✓	✓

AHF = AIDS Healthcare Foundation, Los Angeles, California
CCHER = Center for Community Health, Education, and Research, Dorchester, Massachusetts
EBNHC = East Boston Neighborhood Health Center, East Boston, Massachusetts
Fortune = The Fortune Society, New York, New York
ICAAN = Indiana Community AIDS Action Network, Indianapolis, Indiana
Hopkins = John Hopkins University School of Medicine, Baltimore, Maryland
LSYC = Larkin Street Youth Center, San Francisco, California
MPAS = Michigan Protection and Advocacy Service, Detroit, Michigan
Outreach = Outreach, Inc., Atlanta, Georgia

PROTOTYPES, Los Angles, California
SUNY = Health Science Center at Brooklyn, Brooklyn, New York
UNSOM = University of Nevada School of Medicine, Reno, Nevada
UTHSC = University of Texas Health Science Center at San Antonio, San Antonio, Texas
UVM = University of Vermont & State Agricultural College, Burlington, Vermont
VNAF = Visiting Nurse Association Foundation, Los Angeles, California
HHSCC = Helena Hatch Special Care Center, Washington University, St. Louis, Missouri
WBI = Well-Being Institute, Detroit, Michigan

work due to a disability, 54.2% had a history of problem drinking, 44.9% had a history of crack use, 28.2% had a history of heroin use, 56.9% had reported other illicit drug use, 45.3% had less than a high school education, 49.7% had been involved with the criminal justice system, 20.0% had children requiring care, 22.1% had a history of sex work, 42.9% were sex partners of injection drug users, 46.4% were without stable housing, 11.9% had a primary language other than English and 6.0% were under 21 years of age or over 55 years of age. These characteristics were varied by gender and are shown in Table 3.

Instruments and Indicators

All projects participated in a cross-cutting evaluation of their service activities.[1] A core data collection instrument, *Module 1: Demographics-Contact Form* (Huba, Melchior, Staff of The Measurement Group, & the HRSA SPNS Cooperative Agreement Projects, 1997), was used by all 17 grantees that provided individual client-patient services to collect demographic information. The instrument included items pertinent to describing patient characteristics, as well as major health risk factors.

Using individual data elements, an index was devised (Huba, Melchior, Panter, Smereck, Meredith, Cherin, Richardson-Nassif, German, Rohweder, Brown, McDonald, Kaplan, Stanton, Chase, Jean-Louis, Gallagher, Steinberg, Reis, Mundy, & Larson, 2000) to assess the level of service need or vulnerability. The index included items identified as characteristic of underserved or marginalized groups, as well as items that would impact on service access, understanding of services, and recruitment and retention in services (Shapiro et al., 1999). The index included a set of 15 indicators of service "need" or vulnerability, including being under 21 years of age or over 55 years of age; being a person of color; having a primary language other than English; childcare needs; less than a high school education; being unemployed or disabled; lacking private insurance; having a history of problem alcohol use; heroin use; crack cocaine use; other illicit drug use; having a history of involvement with the criminal justice system; having a history of sex work; being a sex partner of an injection drug user; and unstable housing. Unless otherwise indicated, each need was coded dichotomously, with the need or characteristic being present (1) or not (0). For indicators that were more behavioral in their nature (i.e., substance use, criminal justice system involvement, sex work) a code

TABLE 3. Percentage of Males and Females with Need-Vulnerability Characteristics

	Valid %		Valid n			
	Males	Females	Males	Females	χ^2 (1)	p
Age < 21 or > 55			2579	2225	14.82	< .001
Age 21-55	95.2	92.5				
Age < 21 or > 55	4.8	7.5				
Person of Color			2570	2215	188.75	< .001
Not Person of Color	35.8	18.0				
Person of Color	64.2	82.0				
Primary Language Not English			2343	2180	7.70	< .01
English	89.4	86.7				
Not English	10.6	13.3				
Childcare Needs			1576	1734	453.89	< .001
No Childcare Needs	95.6	65.9				
Childcare Needs	4.4	34.1				
No High School Completion			1422	1675	28.89	< .001
HS Completion	59.9	50.3				
No HS Completion	40.1	49.7				
Unemployed/Disabled			1627	1925	1.62	.203
Employed	13.5	15.0				
Unemployed/Disabled	86.5	85.0				
No Private Insurance			2398	1734	22.23	< .001
Private Insurance	13.1	8.4				
Public/No Insurance	86.9	91.6				
Alcohol Problem			1051	1077	39.32	< .001
No Alcohol Problem	38.9	52.5				
Alcohol Problem	61.1	47.5				
Heroin Use			1054	1061	26.24	< .001
No Heroin Use	66.8	76.8				
Heroin Use	33.2	23.2				
Crack Use			1045	1068	6.29	< .05
No Crack Use	52.3	57.8				
Crack Use	47.7	42.2				
Other Illicit Drug Use			1061	1136	42.72	< .001
No Other Drug Use	36.0	49.8				
Other Drug Use	64.0	50.2				
Criminal Justice System (CJS) Involvement			1126	893	130.83	< .001
No CJS Involvement	39.0	64.6				
CJS Involvement	61.0	35.4				
Sex Work			1027	1098	61.08	< .001
No Sex Work	85.2	71.1				
Sex Work	14.8	28.9				
Sex with Injection Drug User (IDU)			619	878	4.29	< .05
No Sex with IDU	54.0	59.3				
Sex with IDU	46.0	40.7				
Unstable Housing			2062	1836	72.71	< .001
Unstable Housing	47.1	60.8				
Stable Housing	52.9	39.2				

of "1" designated a history of the behavior that had been documented. The composite based on a sum of these indicators could range from 0 to 15.

For the purposes of forming composite scores, complete data for all the indicators were available for a subsample of 2,114 participants.[2] Using the scoring system to index need, males had a mean score of 7.13 (*s.d.* = 2.73, *n* = 1,060), and females had a mean score of 6.75 (*s.d.* = 2.68, *n* = 1,054). The gender difference was a statistically significant, but small, effect ($t(2112) = 3.23$, $p < .001$). Almost all enrollees (87.7%) had four or more need-vulnerability factors.

Procedure

As part of the cross-cutting evaluation effort, individual projects administered Module 1 at program intake or sometimes later in the service episode to update information about the individual's characteristics. Data were typically collected at the individual sites by program staff.[3] Staff representatives from each project received training on the standardized use of the data collection modules at three national steering committee meetings a year for the Cooperative Agreement. Repeated trainings were conducted to account for staff turnover over the course of the project and as refreshers for continuing program staff. The national evaluators were available at all times to answer questions about administration when questions arose. Written instructions for administration were also provided.

Analysis Method

Empirical models of the relationships among the "need-vulnerability" factors were examined using Exhaustive CHAID modeling methods (Chi-squared Automatic Interaction Detector) (Biggs, de Ville, & Suen, 1991; Huba, 2000; Huba, Panter, & Melchior, 2000). CHAID is a regression-type method that allows for a flexible treatment of measurement level for the predictor variables (the 15 need-vulnerability indicators). CHAID relies on an algorithm that works through each predictor variable and the levels of the predictor to identify the predictor that is most associated with the dependent measure–here the total need-vulnerability score–as well as the levels of the predictor variable that most differentiate the need-vulnerability score. Each time a predictor is identified, it is included in a decision-tree graphic that clearly shows the mean score on the need-vulnerability score for each level of the predictor. The algorithm proceeds to find the next most optimal predictor to differentiate total need-vulnerability scores, and so on. The result of the analysis is a set of client groupings representing different combinations of the predictors that maximally differentiate mean need-vulnerability scores.

In these analyses, the minimum final node size was set at 10, and the alpha level of the statistical tests was set at .05, corrected for the number of statistical tests within a predictor using the fairly conservative Bonferroni correction method. All models were estimated using AnswerTree 2.0. The analyses for this paper were planned and conducted between 1998-2000 by Huba, Melchior, and Panter (1998-2000) for the Knowledge Base on HIV/AIDS Care available at *www.The MeasurementGroup.com/KB.htm*.

RESULTS

Figure 1 shows the first two splits in a purely empirical model of the relationships of individual indicators to scores on the overall need-vulnerability index.[4] The average needs and vulnerabilities score for the entire sample of 2,114 clients was 6.94 (s.d. = 2.71). Note that we view this analysis descriptively, not inferentially, because there is a built-in dependency when predicting the needs index from its own components. This analysis is similar to the psychometric goals in scale development when the relations between individual items to their total scale score are examined, and the "influential" items are noted. We use this model to help identify aspects of the need index that are most associated with the global need score. [Technically, the significance tests associated with these predictors would be inflated and should be considered descriptive of importance rather than as formal tests of a null hypothesis (see Huba, Panter, & Melchior, 2000). We do not report significance tests for this reason.] An alternate view of the index components is presented in a later analysis.

Using a purely empirical CHAID model, the sample was first split in terms of the factor that most differentiates participants by their need-vulnerability scores. The factor that produced this split was crack cocaine use. Individuals who were current crack users (in the past 30 days) had higher need-vulnerability scores (mean = 9.38) than did

FIGURE 1. First Two Splits in an Empirical Model of Indicators Comprising Need-Vulnerability Scores in HIV/AIDS Patients

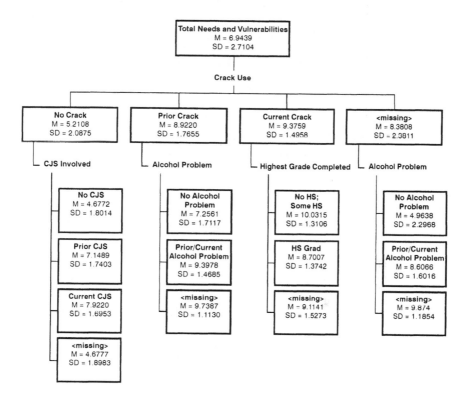

prior crack users (mean = 8.92), non-users (mean = 5.21), or those without data on crack use (mean = 8.38)

Depending on the pattern of crack use, different indicators described the total need-vulnerability scores at the next level in the model. Among HIV/AIDS patients with no history of crack use, total need-vulnerability scores were split by criminal justice system (CJS) involvement. Non-crack users with current CJS involvement had higher mean need-vulnerability scores (mean = 7.92) than did non-crack users with prior CJS involvement (mean = 7.15), no CJS involvement (mean = 4.68), or missing data as to CJS involvement (mean = 4.68). In contrast, need-vulnerability scores among prior crack users were next split by problem alcohol use. Prior crack users with no problem alcohol use had lower need-vulnerability scores (mean = 7.26) than did former crack users with a history of current or prior alcohol abuse (mean = 9.40) or those with missing data as to alcohol abuse (mean = 9.74). Among current crack users, need-vulnerability levels were further predicted by highest level of education: active crack users with less than a high school education had higher need-vulnerability scores (mean = 10.03) than did those who were high school graduates (mean = 8.70) or those with missing data as to highest grade completed (mean = 9.11). Finally, the need-vulnerability scores of patients with no information provided about crack use were differentiated by problem alcohol use. On the average, those individuals who had no history of alcohol problems had lower need-vulnerability scores (mean = 4.96) than did those with a current or prior history of alcohol abuse (mean = 8.61) or those with missing data as to alcohol problems (mean = 9.85).

The empirical CHAID model yielded a set of 31 "terminal nodes"– or independent subsets of individuals with specific combinations of need-vulnerability factors. Overall, the highest need-vulnerability score was obtained by a patient who was a current crack user, had less than a high school education, and had missing data as to heroin use (mean score = 11.38). Aside from this single extreme case, the next highest need-vulnerability levels were obtained by patients who were current crack users with less than a high school education and a current or prior history of heroin use (mean score = 10.84). On the other hand, the lowest need-vulnerability levels in this sample were obtained by patients with no history of crack cocaine use, missing data as to criminal justice system involvement, and no history of alcohol problems (mean score = 3.67). Thus, each of the 31 need-vulnerability combinations (e.g., one need-vulnerability combination is current crack user/ less than a high school education/missing data on heroin use) is associated with an overall need-vulnerability score. A ranking from highest to lowest overall need across each of the 31 different combinations is given in Table 4 under the column labeled "Raw Need-Vulnerability Scores."

As mentioned, the built-in dependency present from predicting total need-vulnerability from its own components represents one way to understand the impact of single elements of the total. An alternate solution is to apply a special "adjustment" to each of the 31 categories of people, depending on the specific need-vulnerability combination. The total need-vulnerability score can be adjusted by subtracting a

TABLE 4. Raw and Adjusted Mean Need-Vulnerability Scores for Terminal Nodes in Empirical Model

Group	Raw Need Score			Adjusted Need Score	
	Mean Need-Vulnerability Score	Rank[a]	Adjustment	Mean Need-Vulnerability Score	Rank[a]
Missing Crack, Missing Alcohol, Person of Color*	10.50	4	−1	9.50	1
Current Crack*, No High School*, Missing Heroin	11.38	1	−2	9.38	2
Prior Crack*, Missing Alcohol	9.74	8	−1	8.74	3
Missing Crack, Missing Alcohol, Caucasian	8.70	14	0	8.70	4
Current Crack*, Missing High School, Current/Prior Heroin*	10.60	3	−2	8.60	5
Missing Crack, Prior/Current Alcohol Problem*, Language not English*	10.20	5	−2	8.20	6
Current Crack*, No High School*, Prior/Current Heroin*	10.84	2	−3	7.84	7
No Crack, Current CJS*, Heroin Missing	8.59	15	−1	7.59	8
Current Crack*, No High School*, No Heroin	9.33	9	−2	7.33	9
Current Crack*, Missing High School, No Heroin	8.31	17	−1	7.31	10
Current Crack*, High School Grad, Missing CJS	8.20	19	−1	7.20	11
Current Crack*, High School Grad, Prior/Current CJS*	9.17	10	2	7.17	12
No Crack, Current CJS*, Prior/Current Heroin*	9.14	11	−2	7.14	13
Prior Crack*, Prior/Current Alcohol*, Prior Heroin*	10.12	6	−3	7.12	14
Prior Crack*, Prior/Current Alcohol*, Missing Heroin	8.95	12	−2	6.95	15
Prior Crack*, Prior/Current Alcohol*, Current Heroin*	9.93	7	−3	6.93	16
Missing Crack, Current/Prior Alcohol Problem*, English	7.81	20	−1	6.81	17
Prior Crack*, Prior/Current Alcohol*, No Heroin	8.75	13	−2	6.75	18
Prior Crack*, No Alcohol, Prior/Current Heroin*	8.45	16	−2	6.45	19
Current Crack*, High School Grad, No CJS	7.28	21	−1	6.28	20
No Crack, Prior CJS*, Prior/Current Heroin*	8.21	18	−2	6.21	21
No Crack, Current CJS*, No Heroin	6.98	22	−1	5.98	22
No Crack, No CJS, Language Missing	5.94	25	0	5.94	23
No Crack, Missing CJS, Missing Alcohol	5.70	27	0	5.70	24
Prior Crack*, No Alcohol, No Heroin	6.43	23	−1	5.43	25
No Crack, Prior CJS*, No Heroin	6.36	24	−1	5.36	26
Missing Crack, No Alcohol	4.96	29	0	4.96	27
No Crack, No CJS, Language not English*	5.76	26	−1	4.76	28
No Crack, Missing CJS, Prior/Current Alcohol*	5.58	28	−1	4.58	29
No Crack, No CJS, English	4.22	30	0	4.22	30
No Crack, Missing CJS, No Alcohol	3.67	31	0	3.67	31

Note. * = Points excluded in adjusted score for these need-vulnerability factors. Each need-vulnerability factor accounts for one point; [a]1 = Highest Mean Need-Vulnerability Level, 31 = Lowest Mean Need-Vulnerability Level point for each need-vulnerability that was also assigned a point in the total score. For example, for the combination in which the participants are current crack users, have less than a high school education, and are missing data on heroin use, two points would be subtracted–one for crack use and another for less than a high school education. This alternate scoring scheme for total need-vulnerability levels describes *additional* needs and vulnerabilities–over and above the needs from the particular combination identified in the CHAID analysis.

Thus, we subtracted one point for each indicator assigned a point in the total. The adjusted need-vulnerability scores for the 31 categories of people identified in the CHAID analysis are given in Table 4 under "Adjusted Need-Vulnerability Scores." The differences between the Raw Need-Vulnerability Scores and the Adjusted Need-Vulnerability Scores can be seen in Table 4.

At the first split in the model, we first subtracted one point from the mean score for those with prior or current crack use (because that is assigned one point in the overall index). We then compare individuals with no crack use (mean = 5.21 additional needs) to prior crack users (mean = 7.92 additional needs) and current crack users (mean = 8.38 additional needs). Using this logic, consider the ranks shown in Table 4. The participant groups with the highest level of need-vulnerability also tend to have the highest level of additional need-vulnerability after this adjustment, although the relative ranks change slightly. A formal comparison of these 31 ranks through nonparametric association coefficients shows very high concordance across the two scoring approaches (Kendall's τ = .74; Spearman's ρ = .89; p < .001). Note that demographic factors (e.g., race-ethnicity) tend to predict additional service needs only after consideration of behavioral indicators such as drug abuse and CJS involvement. However, based on the adjusted need-vulnerability scores, persons of color (African American/Black or Hispanic/Latino) had the highest adjusted scores when data on crack use and problem alcohol use were missing.

DISCUSSION

The SPNS Cooperative Agreement Projects were funded to identify and address the needs of traditionally underserved populations with HIV/AIDS through innovative service delivery models. After five years, the present results support the success of these programs in enrolling these unique and vulnerable populations into healthcare and related services. By any definition, these patients had a multitude of issues and problems that impacted their daily living. As suggested in the CHAID analysis, crack cocaine use, problem alcohol use, education level and criminal justice system involvement were most central in predicting levels of need.

It should be emphasized that the present study is not epidemiological research and the results may not necessarily generalize to all persons living with HIV/AIDS. The Cooperative Agreement Projects targeted populations that were traditionally underserved in healthcare and related service systems. The programs specifically aimed to increase the involvement of high-need and vulnerable populations in care through innovative service models, and projects conducted active outreach efforts to these groups to engage and retain them in care.

Although not every project targeted every vulnerability, all reached highly underserved and disenfranchised populations. In San Francisco, the Larkin Street Youth Center targeted homeless youth and provided both housing and social support to encourage utilization of medical care. Moving clinical care closer to patients in Vermont helped reduce economic and distance barriers for rural patients. In Nevada, the addition of comprehensive nutrition services provided advice and food vouchers to improve nutritional health. For many economically disadvantaged patients, the complexity of completing forms for insurance or for other assistance programs may amplify the barriers to accessing care. At PROTOTYPES WomensLink in Los Angeles, assistance was available to identify and access all needed services including substance abuse treatment and medical care.

Most participants were people of color, who traditionally have less access to care. The present analyses showed that persons of color had significantly greater levels of need-vulnerability in this sample. Cultural and language differences can often increase barriers in traditional care settings. However, many of the Cooperative Agreement Projects specifically addressed these issues with targeted program components. For example, the CCHER project in Boston used a liaison case worker to assist in language translation and interpretation of medical care recommendations for Haitians living with HIV/AIDS. The University of Texas project based in San Antonio had bilingual/bicultural staff to serve the needs of their primarily Spanish-speaking population.

For many patients, current or prior substance abuse was a key issue.

Substance abuse has been linked to a number of areas of concern including retention in care, ability to adhere to complicated medical regimens/treatments, and with criminal justice system involvement. At the Fortune Society in New York City, pre-release counseling and enrollment for prisoners with HIV provided familiarity with services available in the community. Several strategies have been implemented to recruit and retain patients with substance abuse issues. In Los Angeles, the PROTOTYPES WomensLink program serves substance-abusing women by incorporating treatment on-site and linking to a continuum of residential and outpatient treatment resources. The Outreach, Inc. project in Atlanta targets substance abusers with HIV through community outreach. A major goal across many of the Cooperative Agreement Projects is to identify what resources are needed to keep substance abusers in care and to measure outcomes from the provision of these services. Most of these models incorporate or rely heavily on case management and adjunctive services, in addition to access to medical care. The Well-Being Institute serves triply diagnosed women (HIV/AIDS, substance abuse, mental illness) with comprehensive services that utilize nursing case management and onsite substance abuse treatment and psychosocial services. This array of services begins to address daily needs, treatment provision, and assistance in adhering to complicated medical regimens.

The challenge of providing services to high-need patients in managed care environments was explored by a number of projects. In addition to traditional medical services, linkages to adjunctive services through case management in these settings were essential. In East Boston, a community-based clinic providing services to a primarily substance-abusing population used a nurse case management system to organize care. AIDS Healthcare Foundation in Los Angeles provided comprehensive services to an ethnically diverse and geographically dispersed population. Johns Hopkins University created a Medicaid managed care system serving inner-city populations with HIV. For end of life care, needs were met in a managed care system using a transprofessional blended care model by the Visiting Nursing Association Foundation of Los Angeles. Meeting the high needs of these populations within managed care systems required specific changes to traditional managed care and higher levels of reimbursement. Recruitment was often guaranteed by enrollment in Medicaid insurance plans.

Not all of the service models sought to impact these areas with direct clinical services to patients. For example, the SUNY Brooklyn project used training and technical assistance to healthcare professionals to educate providers about state-of-the-art perinatal AZT protocols. Two other projects, based in Michigan and Indiana, aimed to improve access to care for persons with HIV/AIDS by providing legal advocacy and training practitioners in issues related to HIV and discrimination.

Gender Differences

In a comparison of gender differences on the need-vulnerability index, males had slightly higher need scores than did females. This slight difference may reflect the particular characteristics of the patients in these programs, rather than a gender difference generalizable to a larger population. Traditionally, women have reported more difficulty accessing medical care and HIV services. Yet with customized models of care specifically designed to be woman-focused, these programs have been able to increase access for adult and adolescent women living with HIV/AIDS. For example, the program at Washington University in St. Louis improved access for women through combined case management and medical care coordination. Using these mechanisms, access to medical care increased twelve-fold (25 patients in 1995 to over 300 in 1999) and retention in medical care remained over 75%. The program design anticipated the needs of the women upfront by addressing previously reported gender-specific barriers to medical care, such as providing on-site gynecological care and screening for sexually transmitted diseases, women-specific clinic days, on-site child care and the provision of bagged lunches. Program implementation allowed for ongoing barriers to be identified and facilitators of care to be maximized through patient satisfaction surveys, informal focus groups, and a consumer peer program.

Utility of the Need-Vulnerability Index

The index of need-vulnerability presented here is a useful way of evaluating the impact of community programs such as these innovative models of HIV care. By using such a measure in evaluating models of community-based HIV services, it is possible to use the level of need-vulnerability as a key factor in understanding program outcomes such as service utilization, health and psychosocial functioning, and satisfaction with care (Huba, Panter, & Melchior, 2000). By developing a method to quantify level of need, empirical models may be tested so that the nature of these programs and the people they serve can be better understood and replicated in other settings. This index and its relationship to many aspects of service utilization among HIV/AIDS patients have been extensively studied by Huba, Melchior, and Panter (1998-2000).

Grouping of need-vulnerability factors using the CHAID modeling methodology allowed a more intensive look at predicting which combination of needs may require higher levels in intervention. The highest levels of need were seen in substance-abusing, under-educated persons with HIV/AIDS. Looking at these models can influence the level and type of services provided by programs to improve access (identifying that transportation or onsite services are needed) and target service needs (substance abuse treatment or case management, for example). On the other extreme of defining lower levels of need, persons with stable housing and education–probably reflecting employment and higher standards of living–may do better in services relying on more patient autonomy and the ability to navigate a more complicated medical system. Even though the lower levels of need are significantly different from the highest ones observed here, they still indicate several areas of need present that impact on HIV/AIDS care.

There is great importance in understanding the needs of these "invisible" HIV-infected populations to define essential services and examine the way in which they are provided. The SPNS projects were funded to look at innovative ways of addressing these needs in order to increase the number of people served who were previously unserved or unidentified. For these projects, the process of identification as well as the services provided to specific populations were evaluated. Active recruitment through street outreach, linkage of HIV care to other social services, word of mouth, location in areas where the target population lives, pre-release prison planning, advertising, and social service/health department referrals were all methods used by projects to bring in participants. The level of outreach required to get patients into care in these projects helps to illustrate the difficulty of finding the unidentified.

Overall, a major goal of the Cooperative Agreement Projects was to ease access to a wide range of services for underserved groups. There is a need to characterize these populations for planning purposes and to understand linkages among their needs that imply a requirement for additional services. Formal needs assessments were part of many projects, but these primarily informed local program development. The use of a consistent method for identifying service needs and vulnerabilities allowed for a broader interpretation of need to be defined across a variety of populations in diverse geographic areas. The complexity and scope of services available in most of the projects needed to address the needs of the target populations offers insight into necessary linkages, comprehensive services and psychosocial support required to recruit and retain patients in services.

There are policy implications when addressing broader issues of HIV/AIDS care nationwide as the demographic profile of people living with HIV/AIDS changes. The identification of more women, people of color, youth, substance abusers–often coupled with the realities of poverty and homelessness–suggests that new service delivery methods are critically needed to support the expansion of all types of health-related care to serve the infected population (Cunningham et al., 1999). Beyond the provision of medical services, issues of daily living, cultural diversity, addiction, and stigmatization must be addressed to improve health-related outcomes for people living with HIV/AIDS. These innovative projects have collectively described the "invisible" wave of new patients in the HIV/AIDS epidemic. The complexity of the issues these individuals must deal with on a daily basis raises issues about the ability to effectively serve or treat them medically or socially within current care systems.

AUTHOR NOTES

This study was supported in part by Health Resources and Services Administration (HRSA), HIV/AIDS Bureau (HAB), Special Projects of National Significance (SPNS) Grant Number 5 U90 HA 00030 for the work of the Evaluation and Dissemination Center and grants to the individual projects. The article's contents are solely the responsibility of the authors and do not necessarily represent the official view of the funding agency. From the University of Nevada School of Medicine (T. Larson); from Washington University School of Medicine (L. Mundy, K. Meredith); from PROTOTYPES (V. Brown); from the Indiana Community AIDS Action Network (P. Chase); from the University of Washington School of Social Work and the Visiting Nurse Association Foundation (D. Cherin); from The Fortune Society (T. Gallagher); from the University of Texas Health Science Center (V. German); from the Center for Community Health Education and Research (E. Jean-Louis); from the Michigan

Protection and Advocacy Service (J. Kaplan); from Outreach, Inc. (S. McDonald); from AIDS Healthcare Foundation (P. Reis); from the University of Vermont School of Medicine (K. Richardson-Nassif); from the State University New York Health Science Center (C. Rohweder); from the Well-Being Institute (G. Smereck); from the Larkin Street Youth Center (A. Stanton); from the East Boston Neighborhood Health Center (J. Steinberg); from The Measurement Group (L. Melchior, G. Huba); from the University of North Carolina, Chapel Hill and The Measurement Group (A. T. Panter); and from the Health Resources and Services Administration (K. Marconi). The analyses for this paper were planned and conducted between 1998-2000 by Huba, Melchior, and Panter (1998-2000) for the Knowledge Base on HIV/AIDS Care available at *www.TheMeasurementGroup.com/KB.htm*. Special thanks to Rupinder K. Sidhu, Cindy T. Le, Chermeen Elavia, and Kimberly Ishihara for help with manuscript preparation, to Jocelyn Medina and Katherine Ellingson for help with data processing, and to the late Diana E. Brief, PhD, for help with data management, all of The Measurement Group.

NOTES

1. The cross-cutting evaluation was coordinated by The Measurement Group and developed in collaboration with the Cooperative Agreement Projects and HRSA. The evaluation modules are available on the Internet (*www.TheMeasurementGroup.com/ modules.htm*) along with full instructions for their use.

2. The total score was formed for the 2,114 individuals for whom six or fewer of the 15 needs indicators were missing. In forming the total score, missing items were estimated using the EM algorithm. Data from two sites with seven cases each were also omitted when constructing total scores.

3. Human Subjects Protection Committees at each site determined if informed consent for participation in the evaluation was required, or if the data were collected as part of the usual quality improvement process, and hence exempt. Across sites, all data collection was voluntary for clients and providers, so these data have certain non-random patterns of missing observations.

4. Because of space limitations due to printing at this size, the model shown in Figure 1 is limited to the first split. The full color model is available online at *www.TheMeasurementGroup.com/HHC/underserved.htm*.

REFERENCES

Biggs, D., de Ville, B., & Suen, E. (1991). A method of choosing multiway partitions for classification and decision trees. *Journal of Applied Statistics*, 18, 49-62.

Bozzette, S. A., Berry, S. H., Duan, N., Frankel, M. R., Leibowitz, A. A., Lefkowitz, D., Emmons, C. A., Senterfitt, J. W., Berk, M. L., Morton, S. C., & Shapiro, M. F. (1998). The care of HIV-infected adults in the United States: HIV cost and services utilization study consortium. *New England Journal of Medicine*, 339(26), 1897-1904.

Centers for Disease Control and Prevention (1999). *HIV/AIDS Surveillance Report*, *11*(1).

Cunningham, W. E., Anderson, R. M., Katz, M. H., Stein, M. D., Turner, B. J., Crystal, S., Zierler, S., Kuromiya, K., Morton, S. C., St. Clair, P., Bozzette, S. A., & Shapiro, M. F. (1999). The impact of subsistence needs and barriers on access to medical care for persons with human immunodeficiency virus receiving care in the United States. *Medical Care*, *37*(12), 1270-1281.

Huba, G. J. (2001). Introduction: Evaluating HIV/AIDS Treatment Programs for Underserved and Vulnerable Patients, Innovative Methods and Findings. *Home Health Care Services Quarterly: The Journal of Community Care.*

Huba, G. J., Melchior, L. A., & Panter, A. T. (1998-2000). Knowledge Base on HIV/AIDS Care. Online: *www.TheMeasurementGroup.com/KB.htm.*

Huba, G. J., Melchior, L. A., Brown, V. B., Larson, T. A., & Panter, A. T. (Eds.). (2000). Evaluating HIV/AIDS Treatment Programs: Innovative Methods and Findings [Special Issue]. *Drugs & Society*, *16*(1/2).

Huba, G. J., Melchior, L. A., De Veauuse, N., Hillary, K., Singer, B., & Marconi, K. (1998). A national program of AIDS capitated care projects and their evaluation. *Home Health Care Services Quarterly*, *17*(1), 3-30.

Huba, G. J., Melchior, L. A., Panter, A. T., Brown, V. B., & Larson, T. L. (2000). A national program of AIDS care projects and their cross-cutting evaluation: The HRSA SPNS Cooperative Agreements. *Drugs & Society*, *16*(1/2), 5-29.

Huba, G. J., Melchior, L. A., Panter, A. T., Smereck G., Meredith, K., Cherin, D. A., Richardson-Nassif, K., German, V. F., Rohweder, K., Brown, V. B., McDonald, S., Kaplan, J., Stanton, A., Chase, P., Jean-Louis, F., Gallagher, T., Steinberg, J., Reis, P., Mundy, L., & Larson, T. A. (2000). Psychometric scaling of a disenfranchisement index for HIV service need. Manuscript in preparation.

Huba, G. J., Melchior, L. A., Staff of The Measurement Group, & the HRSA SPNS Program Cooperative Agreement Projects (1997). *Module 1: Demographics-Contact Form*. Online: *www.TheMeasurementGroup.com/modules.htm.*

Huba, G. J., Panter, A. T., & Melchior, L. A. (2000). Empirical modeling of patient characteristics and services using sampling partitioning, interaction detection, or classification tree methods: Practical issues and recommendations. Manuscript in preparation.

Shapiro, M. F., Morton, S. C., McCaffrey, D. F., Senterfitt, J. W., Fleishman, J. A., Perlman, J. F., Athey, L. A., Keesey, J. W., Goldman, D. P., Berry, S. H., & Bozzette, S. A. (1999). Variations in the care of HIV-infected adults in the United States: Results from the HIV Cost and Services Utilization Study. *Journal of the American Medical Association*, *281*(24), 2305-2315.

Unmet Needs in Groups of Traditionally Underserved Individuals with HIV/AIDS: Empirical Models

Lisa A. Melchior, PhD
G. J. Huba, PhD
Tracey Gallagher
Eustache Jean-Louis, MD, MPH
Sandra S. McDonald
Geoffrey A. D. Smereck, JD
Victor F. German, MD, PhD
Vivian B. Brown, PhD
A. T. Panter, PhD

SUMMARY. Over the course of the HIV epidemic, the demographics of the populations of affected individuals have changed. Groups that traditionally have been underserved in systems of care have a number of unmet service needs. This article presents results based on data from 478 patients in five national demonstration projects which were funded to enroll individuals from traditionally underserved groups and to help them access services using different strategies. The participants in these programs had a high level of unmet need prior to enrolling in care. Data on client service needs were related to 17 indicators of traditionally

---

Address correspondence to: G. J. Huba, PhD, The Measurement Group, 5811A Uplander Way, Culver City, CA 90230 (E-mail: *ghuba@TheMeasurementGroup. com*).

[Haworth co-indexing entry note]: "Unmet Needs in Groups of Traditionally Underserved Individuals with HIV/AIDS: Empirical Models." Melchior, Lisa A. et al. Co-published simultaneously in *Home Health Care Services Quarterly* (The Haworth Press, Inc.) Vol. 19, No. 1/2, 2001, pp. 29-51; and: *The Next Generation of AIDS Patients: Service Needs and Vulnerabilities* (ed: George J. Huba et al.) The Haworth Press, Inc., 2001, pp. 29-51. Single or multiple copies of this article are available for a fee from The Haworth Document Delivery Service [1-800-342-9678, 9:00 a.m. - 5:00 p.m. (EST). E-mail address: getinfo@haworthpressinc.com].

underserved status including demographic characteristics and risk behaviors, using the data modeling method of Exhaustive CHAID (Chi-
squared Automatic Interaction Detector). Crack cocaine users with
HIV/AIDS were more likely than other patient groups to have unmet
service needs. Patients who were homeless or in precarious housing
also were vulnerable. Results are discussed in terms of designing and
evaluating innovative service models to close these service gaps.
*[Article copies available for a fee from The Haworth Document Delivery
Service: 1-800-342-9678. E-mail address: <getinfo@haworthpressinc.com>
Website: <http://www.HaworthPress.com> © 2001 by The Haworth Press, Inc.
All rights reserved.]*

KEYWORDS. HIV/AIDS, unmet needs, underserved, CHAID

With the changing demographics of AIDS in the last decade, service providers are challenged to reconstruct both the content and context of services and service delivery. Epidemiological trends have
recently shown a disproportionate growth of AIDS cases among Afri-
can-American men and women, Latinas, women and children and drug
users (Carreon & Rodrigues, 1997; Saint, 1996; O'Neill, Talmadge,
Gordon, Gerber, & Sumaya, 1996; Clark et al., 1995; Phillips, Pedreschi, & Cowell, 1995). Racial and ethnic minorities account for about
25 percent of the total U.S. population, but now account for more than
50 percent of all AIDS cases (Centers for Disease Control and Prevention, 1999). As these populations enter the current healthcare delivery
system, services and service delivery processes, initially designed for
Caucasian males with a primary focus on the physiological aspect of
HIV/AIDS, need to expand to provide social and psychological services as part of mainstream care.

In a recent study targeting service needs of HIV-positive women in
the South, more than 300 different unmet needs were identified. The
needs included psychosocial service needs, physical needs, service
and living maintenance needs, and legal needs (Bunting, Bevier, &
Baker, 1999). The medical care needs of women living with HIV are
often complicated and include social and family issues usually not
seen in their male counterparts. For women who see their role as
caregivers first, they may attend to the needs of their family and
partners before seeking care for themselves (Callaway, Brady, Crim, &
Hunkler, 1997). Providers who do not recognize the needs of women
in the configuration and provision of services can contribute to poor

treatment experiences for women and problems in overall adherence to treatment regimens.

> HIV and AIDS-related services built around the model of health-care delivery for gay white males only minimally address the specialized medical and support services required by women. There is a strong need for improved access to comprehensive medical and dental care, child care, respite services, food and nutritional counseling, family assistance, expanded legal planning, transportation and other support services. (Phillips, Pedreschi, & Cowell, 1995)

Similar problems with adherence to treatment when patient needs have not been considered have also been documented in the treatment of HIV patients with histories of drug use. According to Batki and Sorensen (1997), treatment facilities for injection drug users with HIV that provided onsite general medical and social care substantially increased treatment compliance over less full-service programs not as attuned to patient needs.

An extremely high priority in designing services for persons with HIV/AIDS is the development and implementation of a fully integrated continuum of biopsychosocial services. Especially in treating women and children, the provision of HIV/AIDS services framed within family-oriented clinical and support models. Eric et al. (1992) point out that the family clinic model of service delivery is also critical with drug users with AIDS. This population is at high risk for continuing unmet needs unless they can be re-integrated into family networks constructed around them in the service site setting. The creation of a network-like family of services and providers translates to either housing services in one location or making sure that these services are optimally accessible through the ongoing management of a seamless referral system across providers. Building such a system, focusing on the "whole needs" of individuals, can help to improve adherence to treatment and reduce the need for patients to make multiple appointments for care (Clark et al., 1995; Cardona, Mark, Dawes, & Shaker-Irwin, 1995).

An often-missed aspect of service need expressed by women and people of color in treatment for HIV/AIDS is the need for culturally sensitive and competent services. For example, in a study in St. Louis (Scott et al., 1998), HIV patients identified the need for treatment providers to insure that staff composition reflected the demographics of the patients, that there were staff on-site during clinic hours that fluently spoke the patients' language and used culturally appropriate language, and that written materials for use by patients was translated as needed. Similar findings were reported by Ireland and Krauss (1997), who indicated that a primary need for services expressed by women living with HIV was the presence of other women from the community in the clinics and as community outreach workers.

Unmet patient service needs can have a profound impact on treatment adherence. Research indicates that many HIV service providers have not taken into account the need of today's patients for an array of services across biological, psychological and social domains. As the number of people seeking HIV care in the U.S. has grown, the demand has increased not only for medical care, but also a wide range of supportive services (Huba, Melchior, DeVeauuse, Hillary, Singer, & Marconi, 1998; Huba, Melchior, Panter, Brown, & Larson, 2000) aimed at enhancing and promoting adherence to these complex treatment regimens.

INNOVATIVE HIV/AIDS CARE MODELS

In 1994, the HIV/AIDS Bureau of the Healthcare Resources and Services Administration (HRSA) funded 27 Special Projects of National Significance (SPNS) to develop innovative HIV/AIDS service models. Five of the projects focused on innovative medical and healthcare support services provided in community-based or university-based clinics. These projects collected data in common about patient service needs. The five projects are located throughout the United States, focus on somewhat different target populations, and use somewhat different strategies for recruiting and treating patients. Overall, however, each program has tried to address the issues of finding individuals who have not had full access to state-of-the-art medical services and then providing appropriate care. Table 1 gives a brief description of the five projects and their strategies for comprehensive "whole" client care. Additional detail about these program models is given by Brown, Stanton, Smereck, McDonald, Gallagher, Jean-Louis, Hughes, Kemp, Kennedy, and Brief (2000) and by Huba, Melchior, Brown, Larson, and Panter (2000). Issues in evaluating community-

TABLE 1. Five Innovative Models of HIV/AIDS Care

Project	Grant Title	Description
Center for Community Healthcare, Education, and Research (CCHER)/Haitian Community AIDS Outreach Project (Dorchester, Massachusetts)	Enhanced Innovative Community and Hospital-Based Case Management Program	The Center for Community Healthcare, Education and Research/Haitian AIDS Project (CCHER/HAP) of Dorchester, MA seeks to enhance its current community and hospital-based case management system. The enhancement adds one-on-one intensive counseling sessions and educational training to its current system of care. CCHER has developed a Haitian culturally competent risk reduction curriculum. Clients come from the Haitian population residing in the Greater Boston Area who are HIV-positive or have AIDS.
The Fortune Society (New York, New York)	Discharge Planning and Case Management for Latino and Latina Prisoners Who Are HIV-Positive and Symptomatic	The Fortune Society delivers culturally and linguistically appropriate services to Hispanic prisoners and releasees who are HIV-positive and symptomatic in New York City jails and New York state prisons. This project focuses on discharge planning for prisoners, case management referrals with follow-up, and intensive case management post release, including support in making the transition from prison to community. This approach entails identification of and consistent contact with clients prior to release.
Outreach, Inc. (Atlanta, Georgia)	A Safe Place	Outreach, Inc.'s project, A Safe Place, delivers a culturally competent HIV/AIDS intervention model for addicts. Using a peer counselor and street outreach team model for service delivery, Outreach, Inc. expanded enrollment and enhanced retention of substance abusers with HIV by opening a satellite facility and drop-in center within the zip code that represented the highest incidence of HIV disease in the state of Georgia. Activities include assisting addicted HIV-infected clients in obtaining and complying with medical, substance abuse, and mental healthcare treatments. The project also expanded services for individuals who are being discharged from correctional facilities.
University of Texas Healthcare Science Center at San Antonio	Project SALUD	The "Salud y Unidad en la Familia/Healthcare and Unity in the Family" ("SALUD") Project targets the healthcare and human services delivery system for women, children, and their families with HIV in South Texas. Project "SALUD" is a collaborative effort involving the Texas Department of Protective and Regulatory Services (TDPRS) and four Ryan White service providers who have been seminal organizations in the development and delivery of HIV/AIDS services in San Antonio, Corpus Christi and the Lower Rio Grande Valley. This project provides a mechanism for urban and rural communities to build upon existing strengths and capacities for continued development of a comprehensive, family-centered continuum of care for HIV/AIDS women, children and their families.
Well-Being Institute (Detroit, Michigan)	Well-Being Institute Women's Intervention Program	The Well-Being Institute Women's Intervention Program is a comprehensive, nursing-based program designed for substance-abusing women with HIV who are not accessing existing healthcare delivery systems. The program is two-tiered; tier one services assist women in overcoming access barriers to primary healthcare care services; tier two services focus on becoming drug free and providing housing for the women and their children.

based HIV/AIDS programs are discussed by Huba, Brown, Melchior, Hughes, and Panter (2000).

METHOD

Participants

The 478 participants were individuals receiving services at one of five programs funded as HRSA HIV/AIDS Bureau Special Projects of National Significance (SPNS). The sample included 293 males and 185 females. The participants were 59.2 percent African American (16.3 percent of whom were Haitian), 34.3 percent Hispanic/Latino, 6.3 percent Caucasian, and 0.2 percent Asian-Pacific Islander. The criteria for inclusion in these analyses was that the Services Needed and Received measure was administered within 31 days of enrollment to the program so that the measure of unmet needs would reflect the patient's experience prior to receiving services from this program. The mean time from enrollment to administration of the unmet needs assessment was 1.83 days (*s.d.* = 6.20 days).[1]

Instruments and Indicators

As part of their involvement in the Cooperative Agreement, the five projects agreed to participate in a cross-cutting evaluation. The cross-cutting evaluation includes standardized forms used to track activities of individual participants. Sociodemographic data presented here were collected using *Module 1: Demographics-Contact Form* (Huba, Melchior, Staff of The Measurement Group, & the HRSA SPNS Cooperative Agreement Projects, 1997a). Data pertaining to services needed and received were gathered with the *Module 4a: Services Needed and Received* (Huba, Melchior, Staff of The Measurement Group, & the HRSA SPNS Cooperative Agreement Projects, 1997b).

Background characteristics. Module 1 was used to document participant characteristics at program enrollment and to update information as new facts about the individual became available. In the cases where multiple Module 1 forms were available for a participant, the greatest level of risk noted was coded for the present analyses. In addition to demographic characteristics such as gender, age, and ethnicity, a number of behaviors were coded indicating various factors associated with risk for HIV infection and transmission, as well as other measures of need among the HIV patients. A related investigation (Huba, Melchior, Panter, Smereck et al., 2000) developed an index of need-vulnerability for HIV/AIDS patients seen by these service demonstration programs.

Predictors. From the information collected on Module 1, a set of 17 indicators was coded to reflect service needs, vulnerabilities, and demographic characteristics. These variables included Gender (Male, Female); Sexual Orientation (Gay/Lesbian, Bisexual, Heterosexual, Unknown); Age (Less than 21, 21-55, Over 55); Race-Ethnicity (African American/Black, Hispanic/Latino, Caucasian, Combined Small Groups); Primary Language (English, Not English); Childcare Needs (No Childcare Needs, One Child Needs Care, More than One Child Needs Care); Highest Grade Completed (No High School–< 10, Some High School–10-11, High School Grad–12+); Employment Status (Employed, Unemployed, Disabled); Insurance Coverage (Public Insurance, Private Insurance, No Insurance); Problem Alcohol Use (No Alcohol Problem, Prior Alcohol Problem, Current Alcohol Problem); Heroin Use (No Heroin, Prior Heroin, Current Heroin); Crack Cocaine Use (No Crack, Prior Crack, Current Crack); Other Illicit Drug Use (No Other Drug, Prior Other Drug, Current Other Drug); Involvement with the Criminal Justice System (CJS; No CJS, Prior CJS, Current CJS); Sex Work (No Sex Work, Prior Sex Work, Current Sex Work); Sex with an Injection Drug User (IDU; No Sex with IDU, Prior Sex with IDU, Current Sex with IDU); and Housing Status (Own Home, Friend's Home, Unstable Housing). Indicators coded as "current" indicated the risk occurred within 30 days of the assessment, while those coded as "prior" indicated the risk occurred prior to 30 days before assessment, with the most severe level of risk noted during the service episode. Further detail about the derivation of these indicators is available online at *www.TheMeasurementGroup.com/KB.htm* (Huba, Melchior, & Panter, 1998-2000).

Service need indicators. Data regarding service needs were collected using *Module 4a: Services Needed and Received* (Huba, Melchior, Staff of The Measurement Group, & the HRSA SPNS Cooperative Agreement Projects, 1997b). Module 4a was used to document needed and received services in the past six months. A set of 21 service categories were included, ranging from substance abuse treatment to primary and specialty medical care to mental health counseling. The full list of 21 service categories is shown in Table 2. For services needed and those received during the past six months, two composite indicators were formed representing the total number of service types endorsed as needed and received. Individual services were coded as "No, not needed" (0), "Yes, needed" (1), or "Don't Know" (.5). Services received were coded in a parallel way for the types of services received in the six months prior to the assessment. For male and female clients, Table 2 shows the percentage (by gender) of persons who said they did or did not need a specific service and did or did not receive that service in the six months prior to the assessment. Males in the sample reported an average of 8.35 types of service needs (s.d. = 4.10) and females had a mean of 8.99 types of service needs (s.d. = 4.67). The gender difference is not statistically significant, $t(476) = 1.59$, $p > .05$. Males reported receiving an average of 6.77 service types in the past six months (s.d. = 3.82), and females reported an average of 6.83 (s.d. = 4.37), with no statistically significant gender difference, $t(476) = 0.14$, $p > .05$. The potential discrepancy between needing and receiving each type of service was examined using the Wilcoxon signed ranks test. Among males, the differences between needing and receiving services were statistically significant for 19 of the 20 applicable service categories.[2] The one exception for males was needing and receiving inpatient medical services. Among females, there were statistically significant differences between needing and receiving services for 18 of the 21 possible service categories. The exceptions among females were for emergency medical care, HIV-related home care, and HIV-related hospice services. In total, these results demonstrated a high level of unmet service need in this sample.

Procedure

Projects administered Modules 1 (Demographics-Contact Form) and 4b (Services Needed and Received) as part of the cross-cutting national evaluation. In general, Module 1 was administered at client intake, and Module 4b was administered at several times during the course of the service episode. Staff representatives from each project received training on the standardized use of these modules at three national steering committee meetings per year for the Cooperative Agreement. Program staff collected the data. Multiple trainings were conducted to

TABLE 2. Services Needed and Received by HIV/AIDS Patients in the Past Six Months

Needed Service	Percentage of Males			Percentage of Females		
	Received Service			Received Service		
	No	Don't Know	Yes	No	Don't Know	Yes
Drug detoxification or maintenance						
No	76.3%	0.0%	0.0%	75.8%	0.0%	0.6%
Don't Know	0.0%	0.4%	0.0%	0.0%	0.0%	0.0%
Yes	11.3%	0.4%	11.7%	12.7%	0.6%	10.2%
	n = 257, Wilcoxon test *z* = −5.40, *p* < .001			*n* = 157, Wilcoxon test *z* = −4.16, *p* < .001		
Residential drug treatment						
No	65.6%	0.0%	0.4%	73.1%	0.0%	0.6%
Don't Know	0.0%	0.0%	0.0%	0.0%	0.6%	0.0%
Yes	13.0%	0.0%	21.0%	14.4%	0.0%	11.3%
	n = 262, Wilcoxon test *z* = −5.58, *p* < .001			*n* = 160, Wilcoxon test *z* = −4.49, *p* < .001		
Outpatient or day treatment for substance abuse						
No	59.4%	0.4%	1.2%	70.1%	0.0%	1.9%
Don't Know	0.0%	0.0%	0.0%	0.0%	0.6%	0.0%
Yes	18.7%	0.0%	20.3%	13.4	0.0%	14.0
	n = 251, Wilcoxon test *z* = −7.93, *p* < .001			*n* = 157, Wilcoxon test *z* = −3.92, *p* < .001		
Housing or shelter						
No	25.0%	0.0%	15.4%	52.5%	0.0%	2.5%
Don't Know	0.0%	0.0%	0.0%	0.0%	0.0%	0.0%
Yes	7.7%	0.0%	51.8%	14.2%	0.0%	30.9%
	n = 272, Wilcoxon test *z* = −2.65, *p* < .01			*n* = 162, Wilcoxon test *z* = −3.66, *p* < .001		
Food or other basic needs						
No	19.6%	0.0%	15.2%	32.4%	0.0%	2.9%
Don't Know	0.0%	0.0%	0.0%	0.0%	0.0%	0.0%
Yes	4.1%	0.0%	61.1%	11.8%	0.0%	52.9%
	n = 270, Wilcoxon test *z* = −4.16, *p* < .001			*n* = 170, Wilcoxon test *z* = −3.00, *p* < .01		
Dental services						
No	51.1%	0.0%	0.5%	51.3%	0.0%	0.6%
Don't Know	0.0%	1.6%	0.0%	0.0%	0.0%	0.0%
Yes	28.9%	0.0%	17.9%	28.8%	0.0%	19.2%
	n = 190, Wilcoxon test *z* = −7.22, *p* < .001			*n* = 156, Wilcoxon test *z* = −6.49, *p* < .001		
Scheduled outpatient medical services						
No	28.2%	0.5%	0.9%	29.3%	0.0%	1.9%
Don't Know	0.0%	0.0%	0.0%	0.0%	0.0%	0.0%
Yes	20.9%	0.0%	49.5%	12.7%	0.0%	56.1%
	n = 220, Wilcoxon test *z* = −6.35, *p* < .001			*n* = 157, Wilcoxon test *z* = −3.55, *p* < .001		
Emergency room services						
No	78.5%	0.0%	0.0%	69.1%	0.0%	0.7%
Don't Know	0.0%	0.9%	0.0%	0.0%	0.7%	0.0%
Yes	1.9%	0.0%	18.7%	2.0%	0.0%	27.6%
	n = 214, Wilcoxon test *z* = −2.00, *p* < .05			*n* = 152, Wilcoxon test *z* = −1.00, *p* < .05		
Inpatient medical services						
No	71.2%	0.0%	0.5%	70.5%	0.0%	0.0%
Don't Know	0.0%	0.0%	0.0%	0.0%	0.0%	0.0%
Yes	2.3%	0.0%	26.0%	3.2%	0.0%	26.3%
	n = 215, Wilcoxon test *z* = −1.63, *p* < .05			*n* = 156, Wilcoxon test *z* = −2.24, *p* < .05		

TABLE 2 (continued)

Needed Service	Percentage of Males			Percentage of Females		
	Received Service			Received Service		
	No	Don't Know	Yes	No	Don't Know	Yes
HIV-related medical services						
No	8.1%	0.0%	1.5%	14.9%	0.0%	1.1%
Don't Know	0.0%	0.0%	0.0%	0.0%	0.6%	0.0%
Yes	7.7%	0.0%	82.7%	12.1%	0.0%	71.3%
	$n = 272$, Wilcoxon test $z = -3.40$, $p < .001$			$n = 174$, Wilcoxon test $z = -3.96$, $p < .001$		
HIV-related self-care services						
No	58.5%	0.0%	1.1%	61.2%	0.0%	2.4%
Don't Know	0.0%	0.4%	0.0%	0.0%	0.0%	0.0%
Yes	7.2%	0.0%	32.8%	9.1%	0.0%	27.3%
	$n = 265$, Wilcoxon test $z = -3.41$, $p < .001$			$n = 165$, Wilcoxon test $z = -2.52$, $p < .05$		
HIV-related home care services						
No	92.1%	0.0%	0.0%	93.0%	0.0%	0.0%
Don't Know	0.0%	0.0%	0.0%	0.6%	0.6%	0.0%
Yes	4.9%	0.0%	3.0%	1.9%	0.0%	3.8%
	$n = 265$, Wilcoxon test $z = -3.61$, $p < .001$			$n = 158$, Wilcoxon test $z = -1.89$, $p < .05$		
HIV-related hospice						
No	96.6%	0.0%	0.0%	96.2%	0.0%	0.6%
Don't Know	0.0%	0.7%	0.0%	0.0%	0.0%	0.0%
Yes	2.2%	0.0%	0.4%	1.9%	0.0%	1.3%
	$n = 268$, Wilcoxon test $z = -2.45$, $p < .05$			$n = 157$, Wilcoxon test $z = -1.00$, $p < .05$		
Mental health services (inpatient or outpatient)						
No	71.7	0.0%	0.0%	69.0%	0.0%	0.0%
Don't Know	0.0%	0.4%	0.0%	0.0%	0.6%	0.0%
Yes	10.5%	0.0%	17.3%	9.5%	0.6%	20.3%
	$n = 237$, Wilcoxon test $z = -5.00$, $p < .001$			$n = 158$, Wilcoxon test $z = -3.90$, $p < .001$		
Self-help group						
No	37.1%	0.0%	0.8%	51.5%	0.0%	1.2%
Don't Know	0.0%	0.4%	0.0%	0.0%	0.0%	0.0%
Yes	26.6%	0.0%	35.1%	20.9%	0.0%	26.4%
	$n = 259$, Wilcoxon test $z = -7.95$, $p < .001$			$n = 163$, Wilcoxon test $z = -5.33$, $p < .001$		
Family counseling						
No	76.5%	0.0%	0.9%	70.9%	0.0%	0.0%
Don't Know	0.0%	0.4%	0.0%	0.0%	0.0%	0.0%
Yes	11.5%	0.0%	10.6%	17.1%	0.0%	12.0%
	$n = 226$, Wilcoxon test $z = -4.54$, $p < .001$			$n = 158$, Wilcoxon test $z = -5.20$, $p < .001$		
Pharmacy						
No	21.2%	0.0%	1.1%	22.1%	0.0%	0.0%
Don't Know	0.4%	0.4%	0.0%	0.0%	1.2%	0.0%
Yes	5.1%	0.0%	71.8%	6.4%	0.0%	70.3%
	$n = 273$, Wilcoxon test $z = -2.69$, $p < .01$			$n = 172$, Wilcoxon test $z = -3.32$, $p < .001$		
Vocational training						
No	73.6%	0.0%	0.0%	76.8%	0.0%	0.0%
Don't Know	0.0%	0.4%	0.0%	0.0%	0.7%	0.0%
Yes	18.4%	0.0%	7.5%	11.9%	0.0%	10.6%
	$n = 239$, Wilcoxon test $z = -6.63$, $p < .001$			$n = 151$, Wilcoxon test $z = -4.24$, $p < .001$		

TABLE 2 (continued)

Needed Service	Percentage of Males			Percentage of Females		
	Received Service			Received Service		
	No	Don't Know	Yes	No	Don't Know	Yes
Case management						
No	22.9%	0.0%	0.7%	13.8%	0.0%	1.1%
Don't Know	0.0%	0.0%	0.0%	0.0%	0.0%	0.0%
Yes	14.8%	0.4%	61.3%	9.8%	0.0%	75.3%
	$n = 271$, Wilcoxon test $z = -5.87, p < .001$			$n = 174$, Wilcoxon test $z = -3.44, p < .001$		
HIV testing for partner						
No	90.7%	0.0%	0.4%	72.8%	0.0%	0.6%
Don't Know	0.0%	0.4%	0.0%	0.0%	0.6%	0.0%
Yes	3.2%	0.0%	5.2%	4.9%	0.0%	21.0%
	$n = 248$, Wilcoxon test $z = -2.33, p < .05$			$n = 162$, Wilcoxon test $z = -2.33, p < .05$		
Prenatal/pregnancy care						
No	--	--	--	90.8%	0.0%	0.0%
Don't Know	--	--	--	0.0%	0.0%	0.0%
Yes	--	--	--	2.2%	0.0%	7.0%
	N/A			$n = 185$, Wilcoxon test $z = -2.00, p < .05$		

account for turnover in project representatives during the course of the project and to serve as refreshers for continuing staff. The national evaluators were available at all times to answer questions about administration when questions arose, and written instructions for administration were also available.

Analysis Method

The modeling method used in this investigation is Exhaustive CHAID (Chi-squared Automatic Interaction Detector) (Biggs, de Ville, & Suen, 1991; Huba, 2000; Huba, Panter, & Melchior, 2000). CHAID is a method for evaluating regression-type models and is both flexible in its treatment of measurement level of outcomes (such as number of services needed or received) and predictors (such as codes for risk behaviors or demographic characteristics). By means of a systematic algorithm for detecting the strongest associations between predictors and the outcome, a detailed search of the predictor set is conducted. The predictors and levels of predictors out of the entire set that show the most differentiation on the outcome variable are identified sequentially. These variables are assembled in a decision tree format to display the optimally split predictors. Thus, homogenous groups of clients are identified in terms of their observed levels on the outcome measure(s).

In the presented models, the parent node was set at 10 clients, and the child node was set at 5 clients. The alpha level for all statistical tests was .05, corrected for the number of statistical tests within each predictor using a Bonferroni correction. Models were estimated using AnswerTree 2.0. The analyses for this paper were planned and conducted between 1998-2000 by Huba, Melchior, and Panter (1998-2000) for the Knowledge Base on HIV/AIDS Care available at *www.The MeasurementGroup.com/KB.htm.*

RESULTS

Model 1 for Client Service Needs

The first model, shown in Figure 1, uses the dependent measure of total reported service needs in the six months prior to the baseline assessment.[3] The predictor variables in the model were the 17 need-vulnerability-demographic indicators described above. Figure 1 shows the first two splits in the model. The top of the figure shows that for all 478 individuals, the mean number of service needs was 8.60. The

FIGURE 1. First Two Splits in a Fully Empirical Model of Services Needed Prior to Enrollment and Need-Vulnerability-Demographic Factors

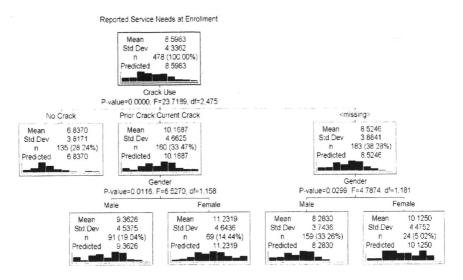

Note. This CHAID model is completely empirical and shows only statistically significant homogenous groups.

graph in the box at the top of the model helps visually show the distribution of the number of service needs in this sample. Because the model that is tested in this analysis is empirical (that is, it is fit to the data using purely mathematical rules rather than guided by theoretical concerns), we can see in the second row of the tree (from the top) what the "best" way is to split the entire sample to differentiate levels of need based on client risk factors. As shown in Figure 1, the optimal way to split the sample is based on crack cocaine use. Individuals who indicated crack use in the past 30 days (Current) or prior to the past 30 days (Prior) reported a mean of 10.17 service needs, compared to a mean of 6.84 service needs for those with no crack use. For those individuals with missing data for (or "unknown") crack cocaine use, the mean number of service needs was 8.52. After considering crack use, the sample then splits by gender for prior and current crack users and those with unknown crack use. Female crack users were further differentiated by criminal justice system involvement.

Model 1 for Client Services Received

The next analysis, similar to the first empirical model, looks at types of services received as reported by participants. The dependent variable is the total number of types of services received by clients in the six months prior to the assessment. This model helps indicate how clients perceive their unmet needs by illustrating the gaps between service needs as shown in Figure 1 and those received (shown here in Figure 2). The optimal way to split this model empirically was by housing status. Clients with unstable housing reported having received significantly more types of services (mean = 7.61) than did those living in their own home (mean = 5.36) or those living in a friend's home (mean = 6.69). Service utilization levels were also relatively high for patients with missing data as to housing status (mean = 7.67). At the second level in this model, service types received were further differentiated for those living some place else other than their own. Among those living in a friend's home, services received were next predicted by use of illicit drugs other than crack or heroin. Active (current) drug users reported the greatest number of service types received (mean = 10.64) compared to those with prior drug users (mean = 6.29), non-drug users (mean = 5.80) and those with missing data as to other illicit drug use (mean = 6.95). In contrast, patients with unstable housing were next differentiated by type of insurance. Clients

FIGURE 2. First Two Splits in a Fully Empirical Model of Services Received Prior to Enrollment and Need-Vulnerability-Demographic Factors

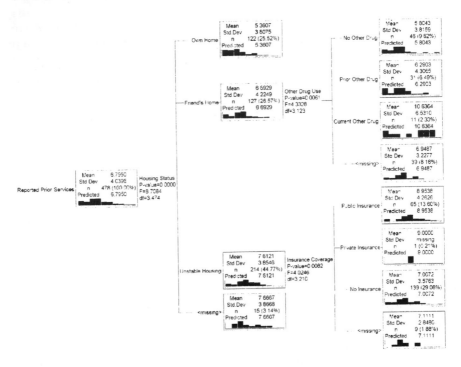

Note. This CHAID model is completely empirical and shows only statistically significant homogenous groups.

with some known form of insurance, public (mean = 8.95) or private (mean = 9.00, *n* = 1) had received more types of services than patients with no insurance (mean = 7.01) or those with missing data as to insurance (mean = 7.11). Finally, the uninsured patients with unstable housing were further split by history of sex with an injection drug user. Those who had engaged in this behavior had received much fewer types of services (mean = 3.22) than did those who did not report this behavior (mean = 7.36) or did those with missing information about this behavior (mean = 7.26).

Model 2 for Client Service Needs (Gender-Specific)

As an alternative to Model 1 shown in Figure 1, Figure 3 shows the first two splits in a model in which the sample was first set to differ-

FIGURE 3. First Two Splits in a Model of Services Needed Prior to Enrollment and Need-Vulnerability-Demographic Factors: First Split on Gender with Subsequent Empirical Model

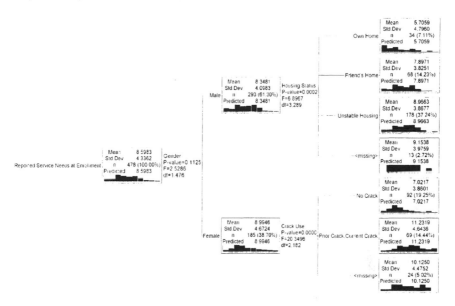

Note. This first gender split in this CHAID model was forced. All subsequent groupings were derived empirically.

entiate service needs based on gender. Following that split, the rest of the model was empirically determined. In terms of the number of service needs at enrollment, gender was not a significant predictor. Following the initial split by gender, males and females do have different factors that predict service needs. For males, those with unstable housing had more service needs (mean = 8.97) compared to those living in a friend's home (mean = 7.90) or their own home (mean = 5.71). In addition, those with unknown housing status had the highest level of service needs identified among males (mean = 9.15). On the other hand, drug use appears to play a larger role in predicting service needs among females. Current or former crack-using females reported an average of 11.23 service needs. These HIV/AIDS patients were further differentiated by criminal justice system involvement, with those currently involved with the CJS having received the greatest number of service types (mean = 15.13). Among females with no history of crack use, those with a history of other illicit drug use had more service needs (mean = 10.75) than did those with no other illicit drug use (mean = 6.67).

Model 2 for Client Services Received (Gender-Specific)

Similar to the Figure 3 model, we also developed a model for services received in which the split at the first level was specified to be gender, with the remaining levels determined empirically. Figure 4 shows the first two splits in this model. Again, gender did not differentiate the number of service types received in the past six months. For males, those who reported unstable housing had received a greater number of service types than their counterparts with stable housing,

FIGURE 4. First Two Splits in a Model of Services Received Prior to Enrollment and Need-Vulnerability-Demographic Factors: First Split on Gender with Subsequent Empirical Model

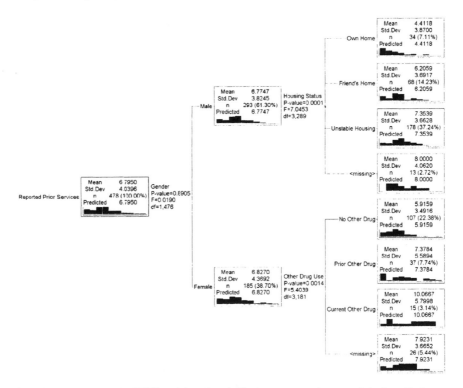

Note. This gender split in this CHAID model was forced. All subsequent groupings were derived empirically.

although males with missing data for housing status had the greatest number of services received (mean = 8.00). In contrast, service utilization among females was predicted by use of illicit drugs (other than crack cocaine or heroin). Current drug users received more types of services (mean = 10.07) than did prior users (mean = 7.38), non-users (mean = 5.92), or those with missing data as to other illicit drug use (mean = 7.92). Current drug users were further split by employment status, with disabled drug abusers receiving the most types of services in the sample (mean = 15.40). Prior drug-using females were also differentiated by housing status, with those in unstable housing receiving more types of services (mean = 12.38) than did former drug-using females with relatively more stable housing (mean = 6.04) or than one female with unknown housing status (mean = 5.00).

Model for Unmet Needs

As a final way to demonstrate the relationship of the need-vulnerability indicators to unmet service needs, we created a difference score between the measures of service types needed and received to form an index to reflect the number of unmet needs that a client experienced. The total unmet needs index score was equal to the number of service types needed minus the number of service types received. Thus, positive numbers indicated unmet needs, zero indicated that the number of unmet needs matched the number of services received, and negative values showed more received services than needed services. Figure 5 shows the first two splits in a fully empirical model using this index as the dependent measure and the 17 need-vulnerability-demographic predictors. At the top of the model, the positive score (mean = 1.80) indicates that participants tended to identify more services needed than what they actually received. The first predictor that differentiated the level of unmet need was crack cocaine use. Participants with crack use in the past 30 days had the greatest level of unmet need in the entire sample (mean = 4.64). The next highest client group was for individuals with prior crack use (mean = 2.41), followed by those with missing data for crack use (mean = 1.33) and non-crack users (mean = .64).

Overall, participants with no crack use reported virtually no unmet need (mean difference score = 0.64). Within this group, however, relatively higher levels of unmet need were predicted by problem alcohol use. Those with no problem alcohol use had a lower unmet needs score (mean = .41) than those with a prior or current alcohol problem (mean =

FIGURE 5. First Two Splits in a Fully Empirical Model of Unmet Service Needs Prior to Enrollment and Need-Vulnerability Factors

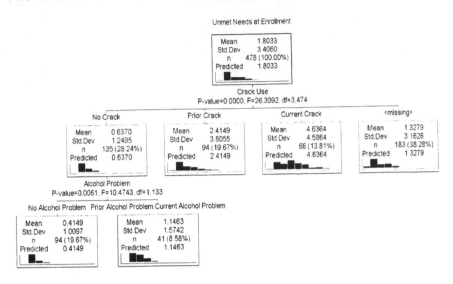

Note. This CHAID model is completely empirical and shows only statistically significant homogenous groups.

1.15). The group with no history of problem alcohol use was further differentiated by race-ethnicity, with African Americans and Caucasians having slightly greater unmet needs scores (mean = .65) than did Hispanic patients in this sample (mean = .10). The African American and Caucasian patients were further differentiated by primary language. Native English speakers had somewhat higher unmet needs scores (mean = 1.29) than did patients whose primary language was not English (mean = .43). In the latter group, unmet need levels were further predicted by education level. Patients with less than a high school education had higher scores (mean = 1.09) than did high school graduates (mean = .14) or those with missing data as to education (mean = .18). Finally, the group with unknown education was split by housing status, although the unmet needs scores in these three groups are close to zero and the cell sizes are relatively small at the bottom of the figure.

DISCUSSION

In this article, a method for differentiating a sample based on a large number of possible predictors was used to study levels of unmet need among participants in five innovative models of care for persons with HIV/AIDS. The results indicated that patients' service needs follow somewhat predictable patterns based on drug use and housing status. Individuals who reported crack use and have unstable housing tend to report the greatest service needs. Gender does not initially differentiate service needs in this sample until other factors, such as drug use and housing, are considered.

It should be noted that although crack cocaine users clearly demonstrated a higher level of service need, they did not show corresponding levels of service utilization in the six months prior to initiating care in one of the five model programs studied here. Thus, crack users represent a group with particularly high levels of unmet need that these programs were faced with addressing. Just as crack users are at high risk for HIV infection, clients who are living with HIV/AIDS appear to be especially at risk for falling through "holes" in the system of care.

Persons with HIV/AIDS who were homeless or precariously housed also demonstrated a high level of service need. This group also reported, on the average, a greater number of service types received prior to enrolling in the model program. However, these numbers mainly reflect the breadth of the services received across different categories. For example, a person who needed housing assistance may still require additional services to stabilize his or her housing. As reported elsewhere (e.g., Huba, Melchior, & Panter, 1998-2000), the need for stable housing among underserved populations of persons with HIV/AIDS has a dramatic impact on their ability to adhere to treatment and on their ultimate health and psychosocial outcomes.

The present results showed that gender was not a statistically significant predictor of the number of service needs. However, it did appear that other factors were gender-dependent. In the models that were purely empirical, gender came into play as a predictor of unmet need only after accounting for issues of housing status, drug abuse, and unemployment. When the models were constrained to consider gender first, however, the relative effects of some of these factors changed (e.g., drug use, unstable housing). Other predictors disappeared from the models altogether (e.g., insurance coverage) when gender was specified first. These findings should be considered in light of targeting services to males or females.

It should be noted that the measures used here of services needed and received primarily assess the breadth of needs across diverse categories. The number of services cited represented the number of services *types* needed or received by the individuals entering these model programs. Patients may have had multiple recurring needs within any given category.

Another caveat for the present study is that the participants were selected specifically because they were members of populations traditionally underserved by the HIV/AIDS services system, and findings will not necessarily generalize to all persons with HIV/AIDS. These findings do suggest, however, that programs that specifically target high need and vulnerable persons with HIV/AIDS are likely to find a number of unmet needs in their treatment population as they enter the system of care. Particularly among persons with HIV/AIDS who are homeless or have a history of crack cocaine use, these unmet needs may be particularly severe.

The present findings reinforced the fact that these innovative models of HIV care were able to engage and retain individuals in care who demonstrated a very high level of unmet need prior to enrolling in these services. Given that reaching the underserved was a primary goal of the overall initiative that funded these programs, it appeared that they were highly successful in meeting this aim. By providing quality, accessible, and culturally appropriate services to these individuals, these innovative models of care served to reduce the gaps in the service system and meet the needs of these highly vulnerable persons living with HIV/AIDS.

AUTHOR NOTES

This study was supported in part by Healthcare Resources and Services Administration (HRSA), HIV/AIDS Bureau (HAB), Special Projects of National Significance (SPNS) Grant Number 5 U90 HA 00030-05 for the work of the Evaluation and Dissemination Center and by grants to the individual projects. This article's contents are solely the responsibility of the authors and do not necessarily represent the official view of the funding agency. From The Measurement Group (L. Melchior, G. Huba), from The Fortune Society (T. Gallagher), from the Center for Community Healthcare Education and Research (E. Jean-Louis), from Outreach, Inc. (S. McDonald), from the Well-Being Institute (G. Smereck), from the University of Texas Healthcare Science Center, San Antonio (V. German), from PROTOTYPES (V. Brown), and from the University of North Carolina, Chapel Hill and The Measurement Group (A. Panter). The analyses for this paper were planned and conducted between 1998-2000 by Huba, Melchior, and Panter (1998-2000) for the Knowledge Base on HIV/AIDS Care available at *www.TheMeasurementGroup.com/KB.htm*. Special thanks to Rupinder K. Sidhu, Cindy T. Le, Chermeen Elavia, and Kimberly Ishihara for help with manuscript preparation, to Jocelyn Medina and Katherine Ellingson for help with data processing, and to the late Diana E. Brief, PhD, for help with data management, all of The Measurement Group.

NOTES

1. Human Subjects Protection Committees at each site determined if informed consent for participation in the evaluation was required, or if the data were collected as part of the usual quality improvement process, and hence exempt. All data collection at all sites was voluntary for clients and providers and, hence, these data do have certain non-random patterns of missing observations.

2. Prenatal services were not applicable for males.

3. Because of space limitations due to printing at this size, the models shown in Figures 1 through 5 are limited to three levels (two splits) each. Supplemental figures showing the models in full color are available online at *www.TheMeasurement Group.com/HHC/unmetneeds.htm*.

REFERENCES

Batki, S., & Sorensen, J. L. (1997). *Systems of care for HIV-infected injection drug users*. Online: *www.hivinsite.ucsf.edu/akb/1997/04idusys/index.html*.

Biggs, D., de Ville, B., & Suen, E. (1991). A method of choosing multiway partitions for classification and decision trees. *Journal of Applied Statistics*, *18*, 49-62.

Brown, V. B., Stanton, A., Smereck, G., McDonald, S., Gallagher, T., Jean-Louis, E., Hughes, C., Kemp, J. W., Kennedy, M., & Brief, D. E. (2000). Lessons learned in reducing barriers to care: Reflections from the community perspective. *Drugs & Society, 16*(1/2), 55-74

Bunting, S. M., Bevier, D. J., & Baker, S. K. (1999). Poor women living with HIV: Self-identified needs. *Journal of Community Healthcare Nursing, 16* (1), 41-52.

Callaway, C. C., Brady, M. T., Crim, L. B., & Hunkler, J. A. (1997). Family-centered care provides women with a one-stop shopping approach. *National Conference on Women & HIV*, 185 (Abstract No. P2.52).

Cardona, L., Mark, L., Dawes, C., & Shaker-Irwin, L. (1995). A community model for an HIV women's care clinic. *HIV Infected Women's Conference*, 119.

Carreon, G., & Rodrigues, A. (1997). WomensCare Center/A work in progress: Looking at women specific services in a male dominated realm. *National Conference on Women & HIV*, 112. (Abstract No. 108.3).

Centers for Disease Control and Prevention (1999). *HIV/AIDS Surveillance Report, 11* (1), 1-44.

Clark, C., Greenblatt, R., Burroughs, J., Dorenbaum, A., Stringari, S., Milliken, N., O'Connor, N., & Jai, N. (1995). Comprehensive specialty-based case in an academic medical center: A model of combined women's and children's care. *HIV Infected Women's Conference*, 98.

Eric, K., Pivinick, A., Jacobson, A., Small, S., Templeton, V., Palmer, V., & Drucker, E. (1992). The women's center: A peer support and family therapy program for HIV infected ex-drug users in the Bronx. *International Conference on AIDS, 8* (2), B155. (Abstract No. PoB 3412).

Huba, G. J. (2001). Introduction: Evaluating HIV/AIDS Treatment Programs for Underserved and Vulnerable Patients, Innovative Methods and Findings. *Home Health Care Services Quarterly: The Journal of Community Care.*

Huba, G. J., Brown, V. B., Melchior, L. A., Hughes, C., & Panter, A. T. (2000). Conceptual issues in implementing and using evaluation in the "real world" setting of a community-based organization for HIV/AIDS services. *Drugs & Society, 16*(1/2), 31-54.

Huba, G. J., Melchior, L. A., Brown, V. B., Larson, T. A., & Panter, A. T. (Eds.). (2000). Evaluating HIV/AIDS Treatment Programs: Innovative Methods and Findings [Special Issue]. *Drugs & Society, 16*(1/2).

Huba, G. J., Melchior, L. A., DeVeauuse, N., Hillary, K., Singer, B., & Marconi, K. (1998). A national program of AIDS capitated care projects and their evaluation. *Home Health Care Services Quarterly, 17*, 3-30.

Huba, G. J., Melchior, L. A., Panter, A. T., Brown, V. B., & Larson, T. L. (2000). A national program of AIDS care projects and their cross-cutting evaluation: The HRSA SPNS Cooperative Agreements. *Drugs & Society, 16*(1/2), 5-29

Huba, G. J., Melchior, L. A., & Panter, A. T. (1998-2000). Knowledge Base on HIV/AIDS Care. Online: *www.TheMeasurementGroup.com/KB.htm.*

Huba, G. J., Melchior, L. A., Panter, A. T., Smereck, G., Meredith, K., Cherin, D. A., Richardson-Nassif, K., German, V. F., Rohweder, C., Brown, V. B., McDonald, S., Kaplan, J., Stanton, A., Chase, P., Jean-Louis, E., Gallagher, T., Steinberg, J., Reis, P., Mundy, L., & Larson, T. A. (2000). Psychometric scaling of a disenfranchisement index for HIV service need. Manuscript in preparation.

Huba, G. J., Melchior, L. A., Staff of The Measurement Group, & the HRSA SPNS Cooperative Agreement Projects. (1997a). *Module 1: Demographics-Contact Form.* Online: *www.TheMeasurementGroup.com/modules.htm.*

Huba, G. J., Melchior, L. A., Staff of The Measurement Group, & the HRSA SPNS Cooperative Agreement Projects. (1997b). *Module 4a: Services Needed and Received.* Online: *www.TheMeasurementGroup.com/modules.htm.*

Huba, G. J., Panter, A. T., & Melchior, L. A. (2000). Empirical modeling of patient characteristics and services using sample partitioning, interaction detection, or classification tree methods: Practical issues and recommendations. Manuscript in preparation.

Ireland, M., & Krauss, B. (1997). Women find their voices: The success of community outreach and case finding. *Nursing & Health Care: Perspectives on Community, 18* (2), 62-67.

O'Neill, J. F., Talmadge, S., Gordon, S., Gerber, R., & Sumaya, C. (1996). Analysis of the U.S. Public Healthcare Service programs to increase access to care and services for women living with HIV/AIDS. *International Conference on AIDS, 11* (1), 394. (Abstract No. Tu.D.2760).

Phillips, R. K., Pedreschi, A., & Cowell, C. (1995). Planning HIV services to meet the growing needs of women in Los Angeles County. *HIV Infected Women's Conference.* P95.

Saint Cyr, M. (1996). Redefining service delivery for women living with HIV. *International Conference on AIDS, 11* (1), 396. (Abstract No. Tu.D.2774).

Scott, K., Gentry, D., Gaebler, C., Myhre, S., Lopez, C., Gantz-McKay, E., & Pasqua, C. (1998). *International Conference on AIDS, 12,* 1072. (Abstract No. 60392).

Perceived Barriers to Receiving HIV Services in Groups of Traditionally Underserved Individuals: Empirical Models

G. J. Huba, PhD
Lisa A. Melchior, PhD
Geoffrey A. D. Smereck, JD
Vivian B. Brown, PhD
Eustache Jean-Louis, MD, MPH
Victor F. German, MD, PhD
Tracey Gallagher
Sandra S. McDonald
Anne Stanton, MSW, CSW
Chi Hughes, MSW
Katherine Marconi, PhD
A. T. Panter, PhD

SUMMARY. Persons living with HIV/AIDS face many issues that make them highly vulnerable to a number of health and social problems. As the demographics of the epidemic have shifted in recent years, many members of traditionally underserved groups have encountered barriers to entering the services system. This article uses data from seven national demonstration projects funded to enroll persons with HIV/AIDS who tend to "fall through the cracks" and help them access

Address correspondence to: G. J. Huba, PhD, The Measurement Group, 5811A Uplander Way, Culver City, CA 90230 (E-mail: *ghuba@TheMeasurementGroup.com*).

[Haworth co-indexing entry note]: "Perceived Barriers to Receiving HIV Services in Groups of Traditionally Underserved Individuals: Empirical Models." Huba, G. J. et al. Co-published simultaneously in *Home Health Care Services Quarterly* (The Haworth Press, Inc.) Vol. 19, No. 1/2, 2001, pp. 53-75; and: *The Next Generation of AIDS Patients: Service Needs and Vulnerabilities* (ed: George J. Huba et al.) The Haworth Press, Inc., 2001, pp. 53-75. Single or multiple copies of this article are available for a fee from The Haworth Document Delivery Service [1-800-342-9678, 9:00 a.m. - 5:00 p.m. (EST). E-mail address: getinfo@haworthpressinc.com].

53

needed services. Data on the initial perceptions of the participants about barriers to accessing services were related to 17 indicators of traditionally underserved status including demographic characteristics and behavioral variables using the data modeling method of Exhaustive CHAID (Chi-squared Automatic Interaction Detector). Through the modeling methods, the groups most likely to experience a large number of barriers to service participation are identified. Having children needing care is particularly predictive of the level of barriers to care. *[Article copies available for a fee from The Haworth Document Delivery Service: 1-800-342-9678. E-mail address: <getinfo@haworthpressinc.com> Website: <http://www.Haworth Press.com>* © *2001 by The Haworth Press, Inc. All rights reserved.]*

KEYWORDS. HIV/AIDS, service barriers, underserved, CHAID

Individuals who have or encounter barriers to obtaining care receive fewer needed medical services and are at risk for worse health outcomes than those individuals with better access. For example, it has been shown that patients living with HIV who lack medical insurance are less likely to receive treatment with AZT than those with insurance (Stein, Piette, & Mor, 1991). Barriers to care extend beyond financial constraints to include cultural, language, and institutional barriers. Those who provide HIV services targeting the general population do not allocate resources to meet the specific language and cultural needs of today's HIV/AIDS patients (Chin, Wong, Chou, Bordador, & Rodriguez, 1998). Disparities in HIV care cut across important population categories, with disadvantaged populations having the least favorable patterns of care (Shapiro et al., 1999).

Demographic characteristics such as gender and ethnicity are associated with disparities in the HIV care system. Piette and colleagues (1993) have found race to be a predictor of unequal access to medical services among HIV-infected individuals, after adjusting for the effects of insurance status and income. The relatively rapid disease progression observed among women may also be the result of unequal access to medical services (Melnick et al., 1994). In addition, an analysis by Hellinger (1993), using data from the AIDS Cost and Service Utilization Survey (ACSUS), showed that after being diagnosed and gaining access to the medical care system, women received fewer medical care services than men, even after controlling for income, race, insurance, and geographic differences. More specifically, women living with AIDS received fewer services than male injection drug users with AIDS, and asymptomatic women were less likely than men to receive AZT.

Substance abuse may also interfere with access independently of demographic and socioeconomic factors (Brunswick, 1991; Kotarba & Williams, 1991; Weissman, Melchior, Huba, Altice et al., 1995; Weissman, Melchior, Huba, Smereck et al., 1995). Drug users are most likely to rely on episodic care, never having received adequate or quality healthcare before their HIV diagnosis (Indyk, London, Tackley, Wennenberg, & Heller, 1998).

Barriers to the provision of care to people with chronic illness exist at multiple levels: the healthcare system, providers-patients, financial-reimbursement, and communities. Enhancement of systems of care, therefore, may require collaborative restructuring across all levels to impact both practice redesign and patient education. As pointed out by Kloser, Ahmad, Parker, and Morris (1993), continuity of care achieved between inpatient and outpatient providers helped reduce patients lost to follow-up; in that urban clinical setting, formalizing collaborative arrangements were instrumental in increasing access to care.

The focus of reorganizing practice involves better meeting the needs of patients who require more time, a broad array of resources, and closer follow-up. Physicians and other care providers need to possess well-developed communication skills, a sensitivity to the needs of diverse populations who may not trust them, knowledge of historical health-seeking behaviors of patients, and knowledge of support systems available in the community (Wagner, Austin, & Von Korff, 1966; Cuthbert-Allman & Chausse, 1996). As Weissman, Melchior, Huba, Smereck, Needle, McCarthy, Jones, Genser, Cottler, Booth, and Altice (1995) report, outreach programs have taught us "critical intervention principles that can be applied to improve access to care for drug-using women." They suggest two key principles to engage and retain women in care: sensitivity to their perceived need and understanding the context of their lives.

As healthcare providers throughout the country struggle to deliver cost-effective and quality healthcare, it is clear that the tension between cost-containment efforts and expanding access to quality healthcare services for high-risk populations may be part of the problem. To avoid unfortunate results, despite well-intentioned efforts, providers must focus services and treatment on the "whole" needs of their patient population. Providers must account for individualized needs;

this focus requires incorporation of a multi-disciplinary team to provide psychological and social support, patient education, and medical management (Sowell, Seals, Moneyham, Guillory, Demi, & Cohen, 1996; Meredith, Delaney, Horgan, Fisher, & Fraser, 1997). The programs described in this article focus on these critical issues in establishing a process to detect, understand, and deal with barriers to both access to care and the continuum of care.

INNOVATIVE HIV/AIDS CARE MODELS

In 1994, the HIV/AIDS Bureau of the Health Resources and Services Administration (HRSA) funded 27 Special Projects of National Significance (SPNS) to develop innovative HIV/AIDS care models (Huba, Melchior, De Veauuse, Hillary, Singer, & Marconi, 1998; Huba, Melchior, Panter, Brown, & Larson, 2000). Seven projects focused on the recruitment of individuals often not linked to the traditional HIV/AIDS service system and the provision of linkages to, as well as supports for, HIV medical care. The seven projects are located throughout the United States, focus on somewhat different target populations, and use somewhat different strategies. Overall, however, each program has tried to address the issues of finding individuals who face many service barriers and to remove these barriers. These programs collected common data elements to measure barriers and facilitators to care. Table 1 gives a brief description of the seven projects and their general strategies for recruiting hard-to-reach populations and reducing barriers to care. Additional information about the model programs is given by Brown, Stanton, Smereck, McDonald, Gallagher, Jean-Louis, Hughes, Kemp, Kennedy, and Brief (2000) and by Huba, Melchior, Brown, Larson, and Panter (2000). See Huba, Brown, Melchior, Hughes, and Panter (2000) for a discussion of issues in evaluating community-based HIV/AIDS programs.

METHOD

Participants

The participants providing data were 519 individuals receiving services at one of seven of the national demonstration projects funded as

TABLE 1. Summaries of Seven Innovative Models of HIV/AIDS Care

Project	Grant Title	Description
Center for Community Health, Education, and Research (CCHER)/Haitian Community AIDS Outreach Project (Dorchester, Massachusetts)	Enhanced Innovative Community and Hospital-Based Case Management Program	The Center for Community Health, Education and Research/Haitian AIDS Project (CCHER/HAP) of Dorchester, Massachusetts seeks to enhance its current community and hospital-based case management system. The enhancement adds one-on-one intensive counseling sessions and educational training to its current system of care. CCHER has developed a Haitian culturally competent risk reduction curriculum. Clients come from the Haitian population residing in the Greater Boston Area who are HIV-positive or have AIDS.
The Fortune Society (New York, New York)	Discharge Planning and Case Management for Latino and Latina Prisoners Who Are HIV-Positive and Symptomatic	The Fortune Society delivers culturally and linguistically appropriate services to Hispanic prisoners and releasees who are HIV-positive and symptomatic in New York City jails and New York state prisons. This project focuses on discharge planning for prisoners, case management referrals with follow-up, and intensive case management post release, including support in making the transition from prison to community. This innovative approach entails identification of and consistent contact with clients prior to release.
Larkin Street Youth Center (San Francisco, California)	HIV Service Delivery Model for Homeless Youth and Young Adults, 16 to 26 Years of Age, with CDC Defined Stage III and IV AIDS	The Larkin Street Youth Center (LSYC) has two primary objectives. First, it has expanded its existing "Aftercare" program services providing emergency housing, comprehensive primary medical care and psychosocial support services for homeless youth living with HIV to serve CDC-defined HIV symptomatic disease or AIDS diagnosed youth. Second, LSYC established an "Assisted Care Facility," consisting of a twelve-unit assisted living and long-term care facility. This permanent housing program is a focal point for providing a coordinated service delivery model that manages the medical, substance abuse, and mental health treatment needs of these young people. The cadre of services provided includes: 1) Social Services–case management, mental health and psychiatric care, counseling, advocacy; 2) Health Services–direct provision of HIV primary healthcare, TB screening, nutrition counseling; 3) Personal Care Services–nutrition, food vouchers, clothing, transportation; and 4) Recreation and Social Activities. This facility is open and supervised 24 hours a day.
Outreach, Inc. (Atlanta, Georgia)	A Safe Place	Outreach, Inc.'s project, A Safe Place, delivers a culturally competent HIV/AIDS intervention model for addicts. Using a peer counselor and street outreach team model for service delivery, Outreach, Inc. expanded enrollment and enhanced retention of substance abusers with HIV by opening a satellite facility and drop-in center within the zip code that represented the highest incidence of HIV disease in the state of Georgia. Activities include assisting addicted HIV-infected clients in obtaining and complying with medical, substance abuse, and mental health treatments. The project also expanded services for individuals who are being discharged from correctional facilities.

TABLE 1 (continued)

Project	Grant Title	Description
PROTOTYPES (Culver City, California)	PROTOTYPES WomensLink: Reduction of Barriers to HIV/AIDS Care	PROTOTYPES heads a consortium of Los Angeles County agencies designed to be a community-based, outpatient (settlement-house) model for delivering a comprehensive continuum of services for women living with HIV/AIDS. Women are recruited throughout Los Angeles County to: 1) provide a range of quality services to substance-abusing women with HIV designed to increase use of healthcare services and adherence to treatment; 2) change risk behaviors; 3) increase compliance with medical treatment and enhance access to existing services through outreach; 4) improve quality of life through comprehensive case management; 5) increase providers' knowledge, receptiveness and skill in treatment of women substance abusers living with HIV; 6) develop and evaluate models for replication and integration into HIV/AIDS delivery systems for women; and 7) disseminate information about successful service models.
Well-Being Institute (Detroit, Michigan)	Well-Being Institute Women's Intervention Program	The Well-Being Institute Women's Intervention Program is a comprehensive, nursing-based intervention program designed for substance-abusing women with HIV who are not accessing existing health delivery systems. The program is two-tiered: tier one services assist women in overcoming access barriers to primary healthcare services; tier two services focus on becoming drug free and providing housing for the women and their children.
University of Texas Health Science Center at San Antonio (San Antonio, Texas)	SPNS Family Unit Project for South Texas (Project SALUD)	The project provides a mechanism for urban and rural communities to build upon existing strengths and capacities for continued development of a comprehensive, family-centered continuum of care for HIV/AIDS women, children and their families living in South Texas.

HRSA HIV/AIDS Bureau Special Projects of National Significance (SPNS). All participants were living with HIV/AIDS. Of the 133 males, 80.5 percent were African American (20.6 percent of whom were Haitian), 12.0 percent were Hispanic/Latino, 6.0 percent were Caucasian, and 1.5 percent were Asian-Pacific Islander. Of the 386 females, 53.1 percent were African American (14.1 percent of whom were Haitian), 29.5 percent were Hispanic/Latina, 15.3 percent were Caucasian, 1.0 percent were Asian-Pacific Islander, and 1.0 percent were Native American. The sample was selected to include individuals who had completed the barriers assessment within 90 days of enrollment to the project.

Instruments and Indicators

As part of their involvement in the cooperative agreement, the seven projects agreed to participate in a cross-cutting evaluation. The cross-cutting evaluation includes standardized forms used to track activities of individual participants. Sociodemographic data were collected using the *Module 1: Demographics-Contact Form* (Huba, Melchior, Staff of The Measurement Group, & the HRSA SPNS Cooperative Agreement Projects, 1997a). Data pertaining to barriers to care were gathered with the *Module 4b: Barriers and Facilitators Form* (Huba, Melchior, Staff of The Measurement Group, & the HRSA SPNS Cooperative Agreement Projects, 1997b).

Demographic Characteristics. Participant demographics were collected using *Module 1: Demographics-Contact Form* (Huba, Melchior, Staff of The Measurement Group, & the HRSA SPNS Cooperative Agreement Projects, 1997a). Module 1 was used to document participant characteristics at program enrollment and to update information periodically as new facts about the individual became available. The measure is available on the Internet at *www.TheMeasurementGroup. com/modules.htm.*

Service Barriers and Facilitators Questionnaire. The Service Barriers and Facilitators Questionnaire (SBFQ) is a 28-item instrument used to measure perceived barriers to obtaining services and facilitators for receiving services. The SBFQ is also known as Module 4b (Huba, Melchior, Staff of The Measurement Group, & the HRSA SPNS Cooperative Agreement Projects, 1997b) in the cross-cutting evaluation of the seven projects. The SBFQ includes 17 items about service barriers and 11 about service facilitators. However, only barriers are considered in this investigation. In cases where multiple barrier questionnaires (Module 4b) were obtained for a given client, the first barrier assessment was used as the data in analyses. Each barrier is scored on a scale of 0 (is not a barrier) to 1 (is a barrier); a score of .5 means that the participant did not know if the item was a barrier.

Total barriers were indexed by a summary score of all 17 barriers to services. These barriers are: thinking the services didn't exist, not knowing where to get services, thinking there would be a long wait to get services, thinking the services were not affordable, believing the client was not eligible to get free services, concern about discrimination by service providers, having transportation difficulties, having childcare responsibilities, concern about disclosure of the clients' HIV status, fear of being refused treatment, concern over losing child custody, worry about being forced to take medication, difficulties making or keeping appointments, concern over language barriers, difficulty communicating the clients' needs, concern over disapproval from family/friends, and caregiver responsibilities. The total barrier scores ranged from 0 to 17.[1] On the barriers composite, males had a mean score of 3.95 barriers (s.d. = 2.96) and females had a mean score of 4.70 barriers (standard deviation = 3.45), with the gender difference being statistically significant ($t(517) = 2.26$, $p < .05$), but small.[2]

Predictors. From the information collected on Module 1, a set of indicators was identified to reflect service needs, vulnerabilities, and demographic characteristics. These 17 variables included Gender (Male, Female), Sexual Orientation (Gay/Lesbian, Bisexual, Heterosexual, Unknown); Age (Less than 21, 21-55, Over 55); Race-Ethnicity (African American/Black, Hispanic/Latino, Caucasian, Combined Small Groups); Primary Language (English, Not English); Childcare Needs (No Childcare Needs, One Child Needs Care, More than One Child Needs Care); Highest Grade Completed (No High School-< 10, Some High School-10-11, High School Grad-12+); Employment Status (Employed, Unemployed, Disabled); Insurance Coverage (Public Insurance, Private Insurance, No Insurance); Problem Alcohol Use (No Alcohol Problem, Prior Alcohol Problem, Current Alcohol Problem); Heroin Use (No Heroin, Prior Heroin, Current Heroin); Crack Cocaine Use (No Crack, Prior Crack, Current Crack); Other Illicit Drug Use (No Other Drug, Prior Other Drug, Current Other Drug); Involvement with the Criminal Justice System (CJS; No CJS, Prior CJS, Current CJS); Sex Work (No Sex Work, Prior Sex Work, Current

Sex Work); Sex with an Injection Drug User (IDU; No Sex with IDU, Prior Sex with IDU, Current Sex with IDU); and Housing Status (Own Home, Friend's Home, Unstable Housing). Indicators coded as "current" indicated the risk occurred within 30 days of the assessment, while those coded as "prior" indicated the risk occurred prior to 30 days before assessment, with the most severe level of risk noted during the service episode. Further detail about the derivation of these indicators is available online at *www.TheMeasurementGroup.com/KB. htm* (Huba, Melchior, & Panter, 1998-2000).

Procedure

Projects participating in the cross-cutting evaluation effort were trained in the administration of Modules 1 (Demographics-Contact Form) and 4B (the Service Barriers and Facilitators Questionnaire) during national steering committee meetings held three times a year. Data were usually collected by program staff at the individual project sites. Project staff members were instructed to administer Module 1 at client intake and to administer Module 4b during the course of the client's service episode. Barrier analyses for these analyses are based on the first time that the client was asked about their perceptions of barriers to service. Trainings on the administration of these modules were repeated to account for turnover in project representatives during the course of the national evaluation. The national evaluators made themselves available to provide update trainings and to answer questions about module administration when questions arose. Detailed, written instructions for administration were also provided.

Analysis Method

To examine how the need variables predicted the barrier outcome, a modeling method called Exhaustive CHAID (Chi-squared Automatic Interaction Detector) was used (Biggs, de Ville, & Suen, 1991; Huba, 2000; Huba, Panter, & Melchior, 2000). CHAID is a regression-type method that allows for a flexible treatment of measurement level for the predictor variables (the 17 need-vulnerability-demographic indicators). To estimate the models, the final node size was set to 10 and the alpha level for each test was set to .05. Note that the alpha level was corrected for the possible combinations within levels of each predictor.

Models were estimated using AnswerTree 2.0. The analyses for this article were planned and conducted between 1998-2000 by Huba, Melchior, and Panter (1998-2000) for the Knowledge Base on HIV/AIDS care available at *www.TheMeasurementGroup.com/KB.htm*.

RESULTS

Perceived Barriers at Initial Assessment

Figure 1 shows the percentage of males and females in the sample reporting each of the 17 barriers. The percentage shown is that reflecting the "yes" responses, or those indicating the problem was a "definite" barrier.

Figure 2 shows the percentage of males and females reporting whether each barrier was either "definite" or "possible." Nonparametric tests for the two independent samples indicated that there were gender differences for five of the 17 barriers, with females more frequently endorsing the item as a barrier. Specific barriers demonstrating statistically significant gender differences include having to wait too long ($z = -2.47, p < .02$); worrying that treatment would be denied ($z = -3.23, p < .001$); fearing that the individual might lose child custody ($z = -2.45, p < .02$); thinking it is hard to make or keep appointments ($z = -3.64, p < .001$); and having trouble communicating one's needs to service providers ($z = -1.97, p < .05$).

Effects of Need-Vulnerability Indicators and Gender on Total Barriers

Table 2 shows the effects of each predictor on total barriers scores. Out of the 17 need-vulnerability-demographic indicators, four significantly predicted total barriers scores. Having childcare needs significantly predicted total barriers scores, with individuals having one child needing care (mean = 5.34) or more than one child needing care (mean = 5.81) having a higher barriers score than individuals with no childcare needs (mean = 4.08) or with missing data on the childcare indicator (mean = 4.25). In addition, individuals with criminal justice system involvement prior to the past 30 days (mean = 3.45) had the lowest average barriers scores, with those with no known criminal

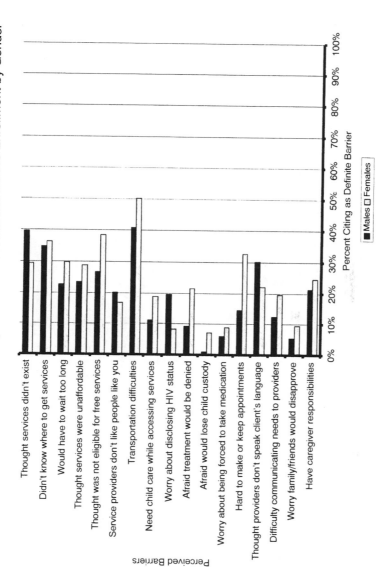

FIGURE 1. Definite Barriers to Care Reported in the Six Months Before Enrollment by Gender

Percent Citing as Definite Barrier

■ Males □ Females

Perceived Barriers

Thought services didn't exist
Didn't know where to get services
Would have to wait too long
Thought services were unaffordable
Thought was not eligible for free services
Service providers don't like people like you
Transportation difficulties
Need child care while accessing services
Worry about disclosing HIV status
Afraid treatment would be denied
Afraid would lose child custody
Worry about being forced to take medication
Hard to make or keep appointments
Thought providers don't speak client's language
Difficulty communicating needs to providers
Worry family/friends would disapprove
Have caregiver responsibilities

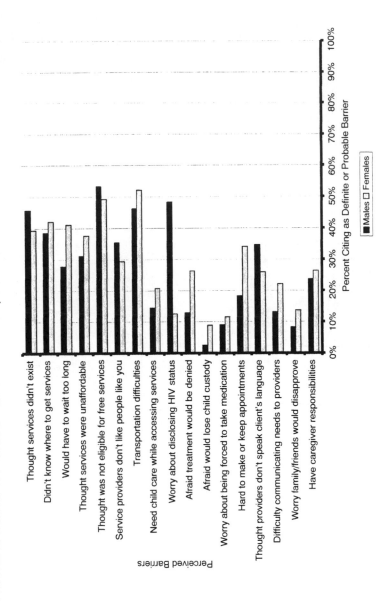

FIGURE 2. Definite or Probable Barriers to Care Reported in the Six Months Before Enrollment by Gender

TABLE 2. Effects of Need-Vulnerability Factors on Total Barriers Score

Indicator	M	SD	n	%	F	df
Age					1.22	2, 516
Age < 21	3.20	2.34	15	2.9		
Age 21-55	4.56	3.37	491	94.6		
Age > 55	4.31	3.33	13	2.5		
Race-Ethnicity					1.68	3, 515
African American/Black	4.32	2.90	312	60.1		
Hispanic/Latino	5.08	4.27	130	25.1		
Caucasian	4.37	3.22	67	12.9		
Combined Small Groups	4.10	3.24	10	1.9		
Language not English					0.73	2, 516
English	4.50	3.24	404	77.8		
Not English	4.50	3.69	112	21.6		
Missing	6.83	4.48	3	0.6		
Childcare needs					7.39**	3, 515
No Childcare Needs	4.08	3.02	328	63.2		
1 Child Needs Care	5.34	3.74	66	12.7		
> 1 Child Needs Care	5.81	3.90	77	14.8		
Missing	4.25	3.31	48	9.3		
Highest Grade Completed					0.85	3, 515
No HS (< Grade 10)	5.01	4.19	93	17.9		
Some HS (Grade 10-11)	4.47	3.36	118	22.7		
HS grad (Grade 12+ or GED)	4.38	3.12	214	41.2		
Missing	4.37	2.86	94	18.1		
Employment Status					0.43	3, 515
Employed	4.19	3.59	56	10.8		
Unemployed	4.49	3.39	267	51.5		
Disabled	4.58	3.18	183	35.3		
Missing	5.27	3.94	13	2.5		
Insurance Coverage					1.46	3, 515
Public Insurance	4.38	3.36	195	37.6		
Private Insurance	3.89	3.50	28	5.4		
No Insurance	4.31	3.43	134	25.8		
Missing	4.94	3.22	162	31.2		
Alcohol Problem					0.23	3, 515
No Alcohol Problem	4.54	3.68	164	31.6		
Prior Alcohol Problem	4.29	3.21	116	22.4		
Current Alcohol Problem	4.65	3.59	73	14.1		
Missing	4.57	2.98	166	32.0		
Heroin Use					0.09	3, 515
No Heroin	4.47	3.51	288	55.5		
Prior Heroin	4.64	3.38	63	12.1		
Current Heroin	4.18	3.06	11	2.1		
Missing	4.56	3.06	157	30.3		
Crack Use					0.20	3, 515
No Crack	4.58	3.78	185	35.7		
Prior Crack	4.39	3.10	125	24.1		
Current Crack	4.26	3.28	48	9.3		
Missing	4.59	3.03	161	31.0		
Other Illicit Drug Use					0.97	3, 515
No Other Drug	4.58	3.51	213	41.0		
Prior Other Drug	4.13	3.34	119	22.9		
Current Other Drug	5.27	4.13	22	4.2		
Missing	4.59	3.01	165	31.8		

TABLE 2 (continued)

Indicator	M	SD	n	%	F	df
Criminal Justice System (CJS) Involved					3.59*	3, 515
No CJS Involvement	4.78	3.64	208	40.1		
Prior CJS Involvement	3.45	2.81	87	16.8		
Current CJS Involvement	4.55	3.39	46	8.9		
Missing	4.70	3.13	178	34.3		
Sex Work					0.65	3, 515
No Sex Work	4.50	3.47	349	67.2		
Prior Sex Work	4.36	3.09	92	17.7		
Current Sex Work	5.79	2.44	12	2.3		
Missing	4.55	3.19	66	12.7		
Sex with Injection Drug User (IDU)					1.66	3, 515
No Sex with IDU	4.17	3.43	223	43.0		
Prior Sex with IDU	4.52	2.92	109	21.0		
Current Sex with IDU	5.08	3.30	13	2.5		
Missing	4.90	3.47	174	33.5		
Housing Status					3.06*	3, 515
Own Home	4.90	3.82	150	28.9		
Friend's Home	3.77	3.17	101	19.5		
Unstable Housing	4.24	3.02	118	22.7		
Missing	4.83	3.12	150	28.9		
Sexual Orientation					2.14	3, 515
Gay/Lesbian	3.58	2.57	51	9.8		
Bisexual	5.48	4.55	24	4.6		
Heterosexual	4.58	3.34	429	82.7		
Unknown	4.10	3.21	15	2.9		
Gender					5.11*	1, 517
Male	3.95	2.96	133	25.6		
Female	4.70	3.45	386	74.4		

Note. $*p < .05$, $**p < .01$, $***p < .001$; "Prior" denotes the behavior occurred prior to the past 30 days; "Current" denotes the behavior occurred within the past 30 days. Percents may not total to 100 within a category due to rounding.

justice system involvement having the highest average barriers score in this sample (mean = 4.87). Endorsement of the fewest barriers was associated with staying at a friend's home (mean = 3.77), whereas more barriers were associated with having unstable housing (mean = 4.24), having missing data as to housing status (mean = 4.83), and staying in one's own home (mean = 4.90). Finally, female HIV/AIDS patients had higher barriers scores (mean = 4.70) than male HIV/AIDS patients (mean = 3.95).

Model 1 for Initial Barriers

The first CHAID model, for which the first split is shown in Figure 3, uses the dependent measure of total barriers to services cited.[3] The box at the top of the figure shows the distribution for the outcome

FIGURE 3. First Split in a Fully Empirical Model of Perceived Barriers to Care and Need-Vulnerability-Demographic Factors

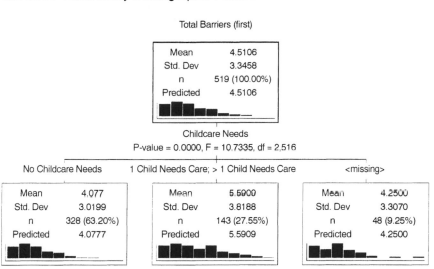

variable, the mean barrier score in the sample of 519 individuals (mean = 4.51 barriers). This empirical model relies on statistical algorithms and identified the optimal predictor from the set to be childcare. The distinction between different childcare situations (needing no childcare, having one child needing care, having more than one child needing care, and having missing data for this variable) is described in the statistical test and by inspecting the mean barrier scores for each of the different groups. Consistent with the simple analysis of childcare needs presented in the prior section, participants with no childcare needs endorsed fewer barriers (mean = 4.08) compared to those needing childcare (mean = 5.59) and those with missing data as to childcare needs (mean = 4.25), $F(2,516) = 10.73, p < .0001$.

At the next level in the model, barriers scores split differently depending on childcare needs. Among participants with no childcare needs, barriers scores were differentiated by reports of having sex with an IDU. Individuals who had not had sex with an IDU endorsed fewer barriers (mean = 3.42) compared to those with a prior or current history of sex with an IDU (mean = 4.30), or those with missing data as to sex with an IDU (mean = 4.51), $F(2,325) = 4.34, p < .05$. Among respondents with one or more children needing care, barriers scores were also split based on sex with an IDU. In this group, three individuals noted to have had sex with an IDU in the past 30 days had higher barriers scores (mean = 9.33) than did those with prior or no history of sex with an IDU (mean = 5.15) or those with missing data as to sex with an IDU (mean = 6.60), $F(2,140) = 3.49$, $p < .05$. Finally, among respondents with missing data as to childcare needs, barriers scores were next differentiated by problem alcohol use rather than sex with an IDU. Respondents with current problem alcohol use had the lowest barriers scores in this group (mean = 1.25), while those with missing data as to problem alcohol use had the highest scores (mean = 6.05), $F(3,44) = 4.08$, $p < .05$. The cell sizes are relatively small for that set of mean differences.

Among the respondents with no childcare needs and missing data as to sex with an IDU, the barriers scores were further differentiated by CJS involvement. Those with prior CJS involvement had the lowest barriers scores in the group (mean = 3.10), whereas those with no CJS involvement had the highest barriers scores (mean = 5.80), $F(3,126) = 3.18$, $p < .05$.

Model 2 for Initial Barriers (Gender-Specific)

In examining alternate CHAID models, one theoretically interesting change would be to see how the model differs if the first predictor variable is chosen by the analyst to be gender. After gender is considered, the remaining need-vulnerability predictors could be empirically chosen to be included in the model. Figure 4 shows the first two splits in a model in which the first split was forced to be gender. Males reported fewer barriers (mean = 3.95) compared to females (mean = 4.70), $F(1,517) = 5.11$, $p < .05$. After the initial split by gender, the predictor search algorithm identified additional predictors within the sample of males and within the sample of females that predict barriers. The males were not differentiated any further in their barriers scores. Females were most differentiated by childcare needs. Women who had children needing care endorsed more barriers (mean = 5.62) than those who did not have children needing care (mean = 4.15) or those with missing data as to childcare needs (mean = 4.49).

After childcare needs, barriers scores were subsequently split by different factors. Among the female HIV/AIDS patients without childcare needs, barrier scores were further predicted by employment status. Females with no childcare needs who were disabled had higher

FIGURE 4. First Two Splits in a Model of Barriers to Care and Need-Vulnerability-Demographic Factors: Gender at First Split with Subsequent Empirical Model

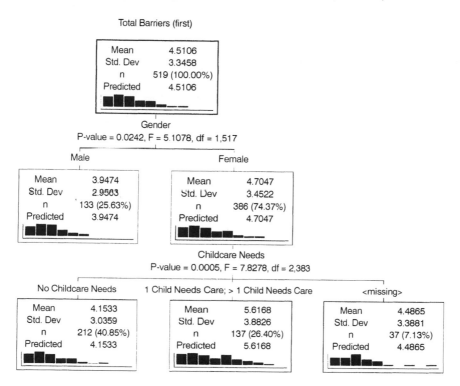

Note. In this model the first level was specified to be gender, and the tree structures after gender were allowed to be fit empirically to the data.

barriers scores (mean = 4.94) than did those who were either employed or unemployed (mean = 3.80) or had missing data as to employment status (mean = 2.33), $F(2, 209) = 3.92$, $p < .05$. Among the females with one or more children needing care, sex with an IDU was the next predictor of barriers scores. Female HIV/AIDS patients in this group had higher barriers scores if they were currently engaging in sex with an IDU (mean = 9.33) than if they had not engaged in this behavior in the past 30 days (the behavior never occurred or occurred prior to the past 30 days, mean = 5.14) or if data as to sex with an IDU were missing (mean = 6.78), $F(2, 134) = 3.72$, $p < .05$. Finally, the barriers scores among females with missing data as to childcare needs were differentiated next by problem alcohol use. In this group, the lowest barriers scores were obtained by females with a current alcohol problem (mean = 1.67), and the highest scores were obtained by those with a prior alcohol problem (mean = 6.72), $F(3, 33)$ = 5.58, $p < .01$.

Model 3 for Initial Barriers (Drug Abuse Status)

In considering barriers to services, drug abusers are often considered to be especially disenfranchised and consequently face significant service barriers. Figure 5 shows a model first split by gender and subsequently split by substance abuse. To conserve space, and because the last split does not yield significant differences, Figure 5 omits the descriptive statistics for each of the groups shown; a supplemental figure, including descriptive statistics for the full model, is available online at *www.TheMeasurementGroup.com/HHC/barriers.htm*. As can be seen, after initially splitting the sample by gender, we found that further differentiating male and female HIV/AIDS patients based on drug abuse history (no use, use prior to the past 30 days, current use–within the past 30 days, missing data) did not significantly differentiate the overall sample in terms of barriers scores. Note that this same nonsignificant pattern was found when we considered use of

FIGURE 5. An Alternate Model of the Relationship of Needs Indicators to Total Barriers at Baseline Assessment, Split on Gender and Drug Abuse

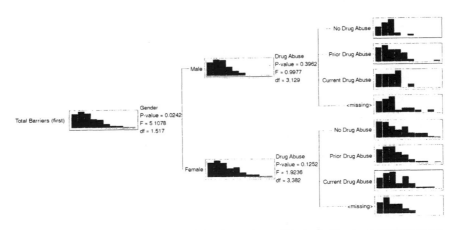

Note. In this model the first level was specified to be gender, and the second level was specified as the composite indicator of whether the participant abused drugs. Note that while there is a significant gender difference, for each gender there is not a significant difference based on drug abuse history.

specific drugs (heroin, crack, other illicit drugs), as well as the more global indicator of any drug use.

DISCUSSION

This article examines the relationships between a large number of need-vulnerability predictors and scores on a measure of barriers that an individual had experienced in attempting to access HIV/AIDS services. Using a purely empirical model, higher levels of barriers were experienced by individuals who had children needing care while they obtained their own HIV services. As also seen in a further analysis where the model was first split by gender, the issue of having children needing care was especially critical for females. Drug abuse status was not significantly related to the reported level of service barriers.

Participants in this study were selected specifically because they were members of populations traditionally underserved by the HIV/AIDS services system. This investigation was not intended to be epidemiological research, and the present findings may not necessarily generalize to all persons with HIV/AIDS. These findings do suggest, however, that programs that specifically target high need and vulnerable persons with HIV/AIDS are likely to find that their clients have previously experienced a number of barriers to accessing needed services. Particularly among persons with HIV/AIDS who have children needing care, these barriers may be particularly extensive.

It should also be noted that the models presented here do not specifically include effects due to site-specific program variations. Particularly with respect to gender, two of the seven programs studied have woman-specific service models and only treat women. Differences based on the other predictors of total barriers scores should be interpreted within this context. Among these seven model programs, the target groups included women, youth, criminal justice populations, and members of various ethnic-cultural groups. Yet despite these differences, all seven programs specifically sought to reduce barriers to care for groups who traditionally had limited access to quality services. The present findings suggest that these programs were indeed successful in reaching individuals who had experienced numerous barriers to care.

The present study demonstrated that males and females with HIV/AIDS had encountered a number of barriers to care prior to enrolling in these innovative services. However, in a number of instances, females reported a higher level of barriers to care than did males. Females endorsed five of the 17 individual barriers more frequently than males. Although some of these barriers were related to issues generally of concern to women (e.g., childcare and custody issues), others were not obviously gender-linked (e.g., having to wait too long or other treatment-specific concerns). The CHAID models reinforced this pattern. Left to purely empirical criteria, the greatest need-vulnerability predicting the total barrier score was having childcare needs. When the empirical model did not explicitly identify gender as a predictor of the total barriers score, this characteristic was confounded with gender. When explicitly including the effects of gender, as in Model 2, having children needing care still emerged as a major predictor of the total barriers score, but only for females in this sample.

The implications of these findings are clear: programs for persons living with HIV/AIDS–particularly those serving women with HIV/AIDS–must help the client with her/his childcare needs to maximize access to needed services. Many of the model programs included in this study provided childcare as an ancillary service for their clients. Ideally, such programs can offer therapeutic interventions for the children–both HIV infected and affected–while the parent receives services at the same location.

Some types of barriers to care may be more amenable to change than others. Adding program components such as childcare or transportation can objectively address certain tangible barriers to accessing services. Other perceived barriers, such as worry about discrimination, communication difficulties with providers, or impact of seeking care on the clients' interpersonal relationships, may be more difficult to change and require outreach and education to ensure the greatest access to HIV care for those who most need it.

AUTHOR NOTES

This study was supported in part by Health Resources and Services Administration (HRSA), HIV/AIDS Bureau (HAB), Special Projects of National Significance (SPNS) Grant Number 5 U90 HA 00030-05 for the work of the Evaluation and Dissemination Center and by grants to the individual projects. This article's contents are solely the responsibility of the authors and do not necessarily represent the official view of the funding agency. From The Measurement Group (G. Huba, L. Melchior), from the Well-Being Institute (G. Smereck), from PROTOTYPES (V.

Brown, C. Hughes), from the Center for Community Health Education and Research (E. Jean-Louis), from the University of Texas Health Science Center, San Antonio (V. German), from The Fortune Society (T. Gallagher), from Outreach, Inc. (S. McDonald), from Larkin Street Youth Center (A. Stanton), from the University of North Carolina Chapel Hill and The Measurement Group (A. Panter) and from the Health Resources and Services Administration (K. Marconi). The analyses for this paper were planned and conducted between 1998-2000 by Huba, Melchior, and Panter (1998-2000) for the Knowledge Base on HIV/AIDS Care available at *www.The MeasurementGroup.com/KB.htm*. Special thanks to Rupinder K. Sidhu, Cindy T. Le, Chermeen Elavia, and Kimberly Ishihara for help with manuscript preparation, to Jocelyn Medina and Katherine Ellingson for help with data processing, and to the late Diana E. Brief, PhD, for help with data management, all of The Measurement Group.

NOTES

1. Missing data on the Barriers scale were imputed using the EM algorithm if there were four items or fewer missing from the total item set.

2. Human Subjects Protection Committees at each site determined if informed consent for participation in the evaluation was required, or if the data were collected as part of the usual quality improvement process, and hence exempt. All data collection at all sites was voluntary for clients and providers and, hence, these data do have certain non-random patterns of missing observations.

3. Because of space limitations due to printing at this size, the models shown in Figures 3, 4 and 5 are limited to one or two splits each. Supplemental figures showing the complete models in full color are available online at *www.TheMeasurement Group.com/HHC/barriers.htm*.

REFERENCES

Biggs, D., de Ville, B., & Suen, E. (1991). A method of choosing multiway partitions for classification and decision trees. *Journal of Applied Statistics, 18*, 49-62.

Brown, V. B., Stanton, A., Smereck, G., McDonald, S., Gallagher, T., Jean-Louis, E., Hughes, C., Kemp, J. W., Kennedy, M., & Brief, D. E. (2000). Lessons learned in reducing barriers to care: Reflections from the community perspective. *Drugs & Society, 16*(1/2), 55-74.

Brunswick, A. F. (1991). Health and substance abuse behavior: The longitudinal Harlem Health Study. *Journal of Addictive Diseases, 11* (1), 119-137.

Chin, J., Wong, F. Y., Chou, Bordador, N., & Rodriguez, T. R. (1998). Improving access to care for language/cultural/racial minorities. *International Conference on AIDS, 12*, 606. (Abstract No. 32422).

Cuthbert-Allman, C., & Chausse, M. (1996). Crossing cultural barriers to care for people with AIDS. *Caring, 15* (18), 14-8.

Hellinger, F. J. (1993). The use of health services by women with HIV infection. *Health Services Research, 28* (5), 543-561.

Huba, G. J. (2001). Introduction: Evaluating HIV/AIDS Treatment Programs for Underserved and Vulnerable Patients, Innovative Methods and Findings. *Home Health Care Services Quarterly: The Journal of Community Care, 19*(1/2), 1-6.

Huba, G. J., Brown, V. B., Melchior, L. A., Hughes, C., & Panter, A. T. (2000). Conceptual issues in implementing and using evaluation in the "real world" setting of a community-based organization for HIV/AIDS services. *Drugs & Society, 16*(1/2), 31-54.

Huba, G. J., Melchior, L. A., Brown, V. B., Larson, T. A., & Panter, A. T. (Eds.). (2000). Evaluating HIV/AIDS Treatment Programs: Innovative Methods and Findings [Special Issue]. *Drugs & Society, 16*(1/2).

Huba, G. J., Melchior, L. A., De Veauuse, N., Hillary, K., Singer, B., & Marconi, K. (1998). A national program of AIDS capitated care projects and their evaluation. *Home Health Care Services Quarterly, 17*(1), 3-30.

Huba, G. J., Melchior, L. A., & Panter, A. T. (1998-2000). Knowledge Base on HIV/AIDS Care. Online: *www.TheMeasurementGroup.com/KB.htm*.

Huba, G. J., Melchior, L. A., Panter, A. T., Brown, V. B., & Larson, T. L. (2000). A national program of AIDS care projects and their cross-cutting evaluation: The HRSA SPNS Cooperative Agreements. *Drugs & Society, 16*(1/2), 5-29.

Huba, G. J., Melchior, L. A., Staff of The Measurement Group, & the HRSA SPNS Cooperative Agreement Projects. (1997a). *Module 1: Demographics-Contact Form*. Online: *www.TheMeasurementGroup.com/modules.htm*.

Huba, G. J., Melchior, L. A., Staff of The Measurement Group, & the HRSA SPNS Cooperative Agreement Projects (1997b). *Module 4b: Barriers and Facilitators to Care*. Online: *www.TheMeasurementGroup.com/modules.htm*.

Huba, G. J., Panter, A. T., & Melchior, L. A. (2000). Empirical modeling of patient characteristics and services using sample partitioning, interaction detection, or classification tree methods: Practical issues and recommendations. Manuscript in preparation.

Indyk, D., London, K., Tackley, L., Wennenberg, J., & Heller, D. (1998). Innovative model for the provision of HIV primary care to persons otherwise lost to follow-up by traditional medical delivery systems. *International Conference on AIDS, 12*, 836. (Abstract No. 42312).

Kloser, P., Ahmad, D., Parker, C., & Morris, F. (1993). Outreach in an inner-city woman's clinic. *International Conference on AIDS, 9* (2), 868. (Abstract No. 3902).

Kotarba, J. A., & Williams, M. L. (1991). Everyday healthcare activities among women at risk for AIDS. *Community-based AIDS Prevention: Studies of intravenous drug users and their sexual partners*. (DHHS Publication No. ADM 91-1752). Rockville, MD: National Institute of Drug Abuse.

Melnick, S. L., Sherer, R., Louis, T. A. et al. (1994). Survival and disease progression according to gender of patients with HIV infection. *Journal of the American Medical Association, 272* (24), 1915-1921.

Meredith, K., Delaney, J., Horgan, M., Fisher, E., & Fraser, V. (1997). A survey of women with HIV about their expectations for care. *AIDS Care, 9*, (5), 513-522.

Piette, J. D., Mor, V., Mayer, K., Zierler, S., & Watchel, T. (1993). The effect of immune status and race on health service use among people with HIV disease. *American Journal of Public Health, 83* (4), 510-514.

Sowell, R. L., Seals, B., Moneyham, L., Guillory, J., Demi, A., & Cohen, L. (1996). Barriers to health-seeking behaviors for women infected with HIV. *Nursing Connections, 9* (3), 5-17.

Stein, M. D., Piette, J., Mor, V., Watchel, T. J., Fleishman, J., Mayer, K. H., & Carpenter, C. C. (1991). Differences in access to zidovudine (AZT) among symptomatic HIV-infected persons. *Journal of General Internal Medicine, 6* (1), 35-40.

Wagner, E. H., Austin, B. T., & Von Korff, M. (1996). Organizing care for patients with chronic illness. *Milbank Quarterly, 74* (4), 511-544.

Weissman, G., Melchior, L., Huba, G., Altice, F., Booth, R., Cottler, L., Genser, S., Jones, A., McCarthy, S., Needle, R., & Smereck, G. (1995). Women living with substance abuse and HIV disease: Medical care access issues. *Journal of the American Medical Women's Association, 50* (3-4), 115-120.

Weissman, G., Melchior, L., Huba, G., Smereck, G., Needle, R., McCarthy, S., Jones, A., Genser, S., Cottler, L., Booth, R., & Altice, F. (1995). Women living with drug abuse and HIV disease: Drug treatment access and secondary prevention issues. *Journal of Psychoactive Drugs, 27* (4), 401-411.

Satisfaction with Innovative Community and University Health Clinic Programs for Groups of Traditionally Underserved Individuals with HIV/AIDS: Empirical Models

Vivian B. Brown, PhD
G. J. Huba, PhD
Lisa A. Melchior, PhD
Tracey Gallagher
Eustache Jean-Louis, MD, MPH
Sandra S. McDonald
Karen Richardson-Nassif, PhD
Geoffrey A. D. Smereck, JD
Anne Stanton, MSW, CSW
Janine Walker, MPH
Katherine Marconi, PhD
A. T. Panter, PhD
David A. Cherin, PhD

SUMMARY. As the demographics of the populations of affected individuals have changed, systems of care have needed to adapt to be responsive to client needs. This article examines client satisfaction data from seven national demonstration projects funded to enroll individuals from traditionally underserved groups and help them access services

Address correspondence to: G. J. Huba, PhD, The Measurement Group, 5811A Uplander Way, Culver City, CA 90230 (E-mail: *ghuba@TheMeasurementGroup.com*).

[Haworth co-indexing entry note]: "Satisfaction with Innovative Community and University Health Clinic Programs for Groups of Traditionally Underserved Individuals with HIV/AIDS: Empirical Models." Brown, Vivian B. et al. Co-published simultaneously in *Home Health Care Services Quarterly* (The Haworth Press, Inc.) Vol. 19, No. 1/2, 2001, pp. 77-102; and: *The Next Generation of AIDS Patients: Service Needs and Vulnerabilities* (ed: George J. Huba et al.) The Haworth Press, Inc., 2001, pp. 77-102. Single or multiple copies of this article are available for a fee from The Haworth Document Delivery Service [1-800-342-9678, 9:00 a.m. - 5:00 p.m. (EST). E-mail address: getinfo@haworthpressinc.com].

using different strategies. Data on client satisfaction ratings were related to indicators of traditionally underserved status, including demographic characteristics, behaviors, and other risk factors using the data modeling method of Exhaustive CHAID (Chi-squared Automatic Interaction Detector). Client groups that were most likely to experience relatively higher and lower levels of satisfaction with services are identified. Overall, all client groups were highly satisfied with the innovative HIV/AIDS services received. The findings illustrate the success of these innovative HIV care models in being responsive and sensitive to the needs of their target populations. *[Article copies available for a fee from The Haworth Document Delivery Service: 1-800-342-9678. E-mail address: <getinfo@haworthpressinc.com> Website: <http://www.HaworthPress.com> © 2001 by The Haworth Press, Inc. All rights reserved.]*

KEYWORDS. HIV/AIDS, client satisfaction, underserved, CHAID

Client satisfaction has emerged as a central and critically important dimension of service effectiveness for community-based organizations (CBOs) serving the health needs of persons with HIV/AIDS. This dimension becomes particularly important in understanding client experiences with HIV/AIDS service as the demographics of the affected populations have changed over the course of the HIV/AIDS epidemic. Ethnic-cultural minorities, injection drug users, and women have been affected by the epidemic in ever-increasing numbers, and members of these traditionally underserved groups have historically experienced barriers to accessing care and taking full advantage of treatment options. Individual HIV/AIDS care programs, as well as the larger health care system in which they operate, need a clear understanding of the extent to which client populations differentially experience satisfaction with services when receiving HIV/AIDS care.

> Qualitative research found patient-provider relationships are second only to perceived clinician competence in determining satisfaction with care. Adherence to outpatient HIV treatments and their outcomes may be improved if providers understand and monitor quality of care by asking patients to report their satisfaction with the care they receive. (Scott-Lennox, Braun, Morrow, Lawson, Tirelli, Dietrich, Hergenroeder, Kreiswirth, McMeeking, Mullen, & Weiz, 1998)

The Health Resources and Service Administration (HRSA), in providing guidance to its Ryan White CARE Act grantees, recommends that service planning bodies and providers pay careful attention to client satisfaction in the development and implementation of their care delivery systems and service arrangements. Ongoing monitoring of client satisfaction by the providers permits people living with HIV to make direct and meaningful contributions to the development of effective and relevant services (Pounds, Finkelstein, Warfield, & Park, 1998). In their ongoing work with client-centered human service organizations, Rapp and Poertner (1992, 1987; Poertner, 1986) suggest that the most effective way of moving clients to "center stage" in human service organizations is to establish an ongoing client feedback system that solicits clients' perceptions of service satisfaction.

CLIENT SATISFACTION AND SERVICE DELIVERY

Often, the concept of client satisfaction is considered to be an indirect measure or proxy for service quality. Client satisfaction is perceived to relate entirely to a client's perceptions of care and not necessarily to the more concrete outcomes of service. However, satisfaction should be viewed as the client's assessment of the appropriateness of services received and the meaningfulness of the treatment outcomes achieved. Identified as the third critical component of service effectiveness by Patti (1987), along with treatment outcomes and service delivery cost efficiencies, satisfaction provides the most important direct feedback to providers on the quality of their services and the relationship of these services to treatment outcomes. Evaluating client satisfaction permits CBOs to put in context both their service process outputs and their treatment outcomes.

Client satisfaction is an important overall indicator of the clients' perceptions of the "workings" of a CBO and is a reflection of the interaction of the client with the service system. Satisfaction deals specifically with the quality and clarity of communications by providers (e.g., Scott-Lennox et al., 1998), perception of the exchange of services and information from the provider to the client (Powell-Cope, Brown, Holzemer, Corless, Turner, Nokes, & Inouye, 1998; Burke, Cohen, Weber, Garcia, Sha, & Hershow, 1998), and perceived respect from providers, including willingness to answer questions (e.g., Aiken, Sloane, Lake, Sochalski, & Weber, 1999; Huba, Melchior, Staff of The Measurement Group, & the HRSA SPNS Cooperative Agreement Projects 1997a,b).

Overall, satisfaction with services is driven, to a large extent, by the personal perceptions. Given the personal aspect of client satisfaction, it is important for CBOs to design and implement services that recognize the unique social and cultural needs of the clients being served. Johnson (1994) notes that when providers design service settings that reflect the culture of clients being served, clients' satisfaction with services consistently and significantly increases. Similar findings were reported by Rapkin, Smith, Feldman, Cruz, Plavin and Jemiolo (1998) in a study of 992 Medicaid HIV/AIDS patients in treatment in a wide range of service sites in New York City. Strong and positive relationships with providers, defined as a lack of cultural and ethnic discrimination towards clients by providers, were found to be a key in producing higher satisfaction with services by clients. Morrow and Fuqua (1997), in work with HIV/STD prevention training with women who have sex with other women, found that programs that reported the highest level of client satisfaction were programs developed and implemented within client-specific contexts.

CBOs providing HIV/AIDS services need to understand the connection between client satisfaction with services and the clients' continuance with treatment. In addition, CBOs must recognize, that in large part, client satisfaction with treatment is driven by the cultural, social and behavioral contexts in which services are designed and implemented. The critical nature of client satisfaction is especially amplified in today's environment as historically disenfranchised populations form the majority of patients in need of HIV/AIDS treatment and services (Centers for Disease Control and Prevention, 1999).

Given the current demographics of the AIDS epidemic, it is critical that CBOs and full service primary care clinic providers track sociodemographic characteristics of their client population. Analyses of such data are important in describing the configuration of services received and retention of clients in service. Failure to consider sociodemographic profiles of patients and their specific behaviors that impact therapy may result in significant non-adherence with treatment and treatment failures, as reported by Lucas (1999).

INNOVATIVE HIV/AIDS SERVICE MODELS

In 1994, the HIV/AIDS Bureau (HAB) of the Health Resources and Services Administration (HRSA) funded Special Projects of National

Significance (SPNS) to develop innovative HIV/AIDS service models. Seven projects focused on innovative medical and medical support services provided in community-based or university-based clinics. The seven projects are located throughout the United States, focus on somewhat different target populations, and use somewhat different strategies for recruiting and treating patients. Overall, however, each program has tried to address the issues of finding individuals who have not had full access to state-of-the-art medical services and then providing appropriate treatment. Table 1 gives a brief description of the seven projects and their strategies for recruiting hard-to-reach populations and delivering services. The models are described in more detail by Brown, Stanton, Smereck, McDonald, Gallagher, Jean-Louis, Hughes, Kemp, Kennedy, and Brief (2000), Richardson-Nassif, Meredith, Larson, Mundy, and Melchior (2000), and Huba, Melchior, Brown, Larson, and Panter (2000). Issues in evaluating community-based HIV/AIDS programs are discussed by Huba, Brown, Melchior, Hughes, and Panter (2000). Six of the seven projects are Community-Based Organizations (CBOs) providing psychosocial support services to HIV/AIDS clients linked to medical providers, and one project is a comprehensive, university-based medical clinic providing integrated psychosocial supports.

Each program, while incorporating unique and innovative approaches to delivering services in this study, shared three unifying concepts in the development and implementation of its service delivery model. First, each program recognized the connection between client satisfaction with services and sustaining clients in treatment. Second, each program further recognized that satisfaction was strongly dependent on aligning services to the social, cultural and behavioral norms of the populations being treated. Finally, each project incorporated the routine and continuous monitoring of client satisfaction into the implementation of services. Thus, by identifying direct client feedback as a critical service component, these programs were in a position to effectively evaluate their success in implementing client-centered care.

METHOD

Participants

The 516 participants received services at one of seven national demonstration projects funded as part of the HRSA/HAB SPNS Coop-

TABLE 1. Seven SPNS Cooperative Agreement Projects: Project Summaries

Project	Grant Title	Description
Center for Community Health, Education, and Research (CCHER)/Haitian Community AIDS Outreach Project (Dorchester, Massachusetts)	Enhanced Innovative Community and Hospital-Based Case Management Program	The Center for Community Health, Education and Research/Haitian AIDS Project (CCHER/HAP) of Dorchester, Massachusetts seeks to enhance its current community and hospital-based case management system. The enhancement adds one-on-one intensive counseling sessions and educational training to its current system of care. CCHER has developed a Haitian culturally competent risk reduction curriculum. Clients come from the Haitian population residing in the Greater Boston Area who are HIV-positive or have AIDS.
The Fortune Society (New York, New York)	Discharge Planning and Case Management for Latino and Latina Prisoners Who Are HIV-Positive and Symptomatic	The Fortune Society delivers culturally and linguistically appropriate services to Hispanic prisoners and releasees who are HIV-positive and symptomatic in New York City jails and New York state prisons. This project focuses on discharge planning for prisoners, case management referrals with follow-up, and intensive case management post release, including support in making the transition from prison to community. This innovative approach entails identification of and consistent contact with clients prior to release.
Larkin Street Youth Center (San Francisco, California)	HIV Service Delivery Model for Homeless Youth and Young Adults, 16 to 26 Years of Age, with CDC Defined Stage III and IV AIDS	The Larkin Street Youth Center (LSYC) has two primary objectives. First, the program has expanded their existing "Aftercare" program services which provide emergency housing, comprehensive primary medical care and psychosocial support services for homeless youth living with HIV to serve CDC-defined HIV symptomatic disease or AIDS diagnosed youth. Second, LSYC has established an "Assisted Care Facility" consisting of a twelve-unit assisted living and long-term care facility. This permanent housing program is a focal point for providing a coordinated service delivery model that manages the medical, substance abuse, and mental health treatment needs of these young people. The cadre of services provided includes: (1) Social Services–case management, mental health and psychiatric care, counseling, advocacy; (2) Health Services–direct provision of HIV primary health care, TB screening, nutrition counseling; (3) Personal Care Services–nutrition, food vouchers, clothing, transportation; and (4) Recreation and Social Activities. This facility is open and supervised 24 hours a day.

Outreach, Inc. (Atlanta, Georgia)	A Safe Place	Outreach, Inc.'s project, A Safe Place, delivers a culturally competent HIV/AIDS intervention model for addicts. Using a peer counselor and street outreach team model for service delivery, Outreach, Inc. expanded enrollment and enhanced retention of substance abusers with HIV by opening a satellite facility and drop-in center within the zip code that represented the highest incidence of HIV disease in the state of Georgia. Activities include assisting addicted HIV-infected clients in obtaining and complying with medical, substance abuse, and mental health treatments. The project also expanded services for individuals who are being discharged from correctional facilities.
PROTOTYPES (Culver City, California)	PROTOTYPES WomensLink: Reduction of Barriers to HIV/AIDS Care	PROTOTYPES heads a consortium of Los Angeles County agencies designed to be a community-based, outpatient (settlement-house) model for delivering a comprehensive continuum of services for women living with HIV/AIDS. Women are recruited throughout Los Angeles County to: (1) provide a range of quality services to substance-abusing women with HIV designed to increase use of health care services and adherence to treatment; (2) change risk behaviors; (3) increase compliance with medical treatment and enhance access to existing services through outreach; (4) improve quality of life through comprehensive case management; (5) increase providers' knowledge, receptiveness and skill in treatment of women substance abusers living with HIV; (6) develop and evaluate models for replication and integration into HIV/AIDS delivery systems for women; and (7) disseminate information about successful service models.
University of Vermont & State Agricultural College (Burlington, Vermont)	Health Care Delivery for People with HIV/AIDS in Rural Vermont	The project has developed three state-of-the-art rural community HIV satellite clinics in Vermont that supplement services currently being provided by the state's only other comprehensive HIV clinic.
Well-Being Institute (Detroit, Michigan)	Well-Being Institute Women's Intervention Program	The Well-Being Institute Women's Intervention Program is a comprehensive, nursing-based intervention program designed for substance-abusing women with HIV who are not accessing existing health delivery systems. The program is two-tiered: tier one services assist women in overcoming access barriers to primary health care services; tier two services focus on becoming drug free and providing housing for the women and their children.

erative Agreement. All participants were living with HIV/AIDS. The sample was approximately equally comprised of males (48.4 percent) and females (51.6 percent). The participants were 58.9 percent African American (12.8 percent of whom were Haitian), 19.6 percent Hispanic/Latino, 19.6 percent Caucasian, 1.0 percent Asian-Pacific Islander, and 1.0 percent Native American or other ethnicities.

Instruments and Indicators

As part of their involvement in the HRSA SPNS Cooperative Agreement, the seven projects agreed to participate in a cross-cutting evaluation (see Huba, Melchior, De Veauuse, Hillary, Singer, & Marconi, 1998; Huba, Melchior, Panter, Brown, & Larson, 2000). The cross-cutting evaluation includes standardized forms used to track activities of individual participants. Sociodemographic data presented here were collected using *Module 1: Demographics-Contact Form* (Huba, Melchior, Staff of The Measurement Group, & the HRSA SPNS Cooperative Agreement Projects, 1997a). Data pertaining to client satisfaction were gathered with the *Module 11: Client Satisfaction Survey* (Huba, Melchior, Staff of The Measurement Group, & the HRSA SPNS Cooperative Agreement Projects, 1997b).[1]

Background characteristics. Module 1 was the central way that the programs documented participant characteristics at program enrollment. It was also used to update information, as new data about the individual became available. In cases in which multiple Module 1 forms were available for a given participant, the greatest level of risk noted was coded. In addition to demographic characteristics such as gender, age, and ethnicity, a number of behaviors were coded indicating various factors associated with risk for HIV infection and transmission, as well as other measures of need among the HIV patients. A related investigation (Huba, Melchior, Panter, Smereck, Meredith, Cherin, Richardson-Nassif, German, Rohweder, Brown, McDonald, Kaplan, Stanton, Chase, Jean-Louis, Gallagher, Steinberg, Reis, Mundy, & Larson, 2000) developed an index of need-vulnerability for HIV/AIDS patients served by these service demonstration programs. Characteristics such as age, ethnicity, employment status, childcare needs, education level, housing stability, and drug abuse history were studied as factors affecting client satisfaction.

Predictors. From the information collected on Module 1, a set of 17 indicators was coded to reflect service needs, vulnerabilities, and demographic characteristics. These variables included Gender (Male, Female); Sexual Orientation (Gay/Lesbian, Bisexual, Heterosexual, Unknown); Age (Less than 21, 21-55, Over 55); Race-Ethnicity (African American/Black, Hispanic/Latino, Caucasian, Combined Small Groups); Primary Language (English, Not English); Childcare Needs (No Childcare Needs, One Child Needs Care, More than One Child Needs Care); Highest Grade Completed (No High School–< 10, Some High School–10-11, High School Grad–12+); Employment Status (Employed, Unemployed, Disabled); Insurance Coverage (Public Insurance, Private Insurance, No Insurance); Problem Alcohol Use (No Alcohol Problem, Prior Alcohol Problem, Current Alcohol Problem); Heroin Use (No Heroin, Prior Heroin, Current Heroin); Crack Cocaine Use (No Crack, Prior Crack, Current Crack); Other Illicit Drug Use (No Other Drug, Prior Other Drug, Current Other Drug); Involvement with the Criminal Justice System (CJS; No CJS, Prior CJS, Current CJS); Sex Work (No Sex Work, Prior Sex Work, Current Sex Work); Sex with an Injection Drug User (IDU; No Sex with IDU, Prior Sex with IDU, Current Sex with IDU); and Housing Status (Own Home, Friend's Home, Unstable Housing). Indicators coded as "current" indicate the risk occurred within 30 days of the assessment, while those coded as "prior" indicate the risk occurred prior to 30 days before assessment, with the most severe level of risk noted during the service episode. Further detail about the derivation of these indicators is available online at *www.TheMeasurementGroup.com/KB.htm* (Huba, Melchior, & Panter, 1998-2000).

Client satisfaction indicators. Module 11 was used to document ratings of client satisfaction with services and the overall program. The items included ratings of overall services, information provided to clients, staff ability to answer questions, staff ability to explain treatment procedures, staff ability to treat the client as an individual, staff respect of privacy, staff helpfulness, and likelihood to recommend the program to others. For these analyses, two different indices of satisfaction were used.

The first indicator used in the analyses was a single item, four-category rating of overall satisfaction coded as "fair/poor" (1), "good" (2), "very good" (3), or "excellent" (4).

The second indicator was the sum score of eight client satisfaction items (scores range from 8 to 32).[2] The satisfaction ratings that reflected the last time the participant completed Module 11 were included in the analyses. These "final" satisfaction ratings were obtained an average of 536.55 days (s.d. = 372.27 days) from program enrollment, with a range of 61 to 1632 days after enrollment. Table 2 shows the percentage of respondents by gender rating services as either "very good" or "excellent." Note that client satisfaction levels were extremely high for all categories. Overall satisfaction scores did not differ by gender, and category ratings were consistently in the "very good" and "excellent" range (80 percent or higher).

Procedure

As part of the cross-cutting evaluation effort, individual projects administered Modules 1 (Demographics-Contact Form) and 11 (Client Satisfaction). In general, Module 1 was administered at client intake, and Module 11 was administered at several times during the course of the service episode. Staff representatives from each project received training on the standardized use of these modules at three national steering committee meetings a year for the Cooperative Agreement. At the individual project sites, data were typically collected by program staff. Repeated trainings were conducted to account for turnover in project representatives during the course of the project and to serve as refreshers for continuing staff. The national evaluators were available at all times to answer questions about administration when ques-

TABLE 2. Satisfaction Ratings for Males and Females Served by These Seven Projects

	Percentage Among Males (*n* = 250)	Percentage Among Females (*n* = 266)
Services were "excellent" or "very good"	79.8%	81.5%
Information received was "very helpful" or "helpful"	96.2%	97.9%
Staff answered questions "all" or "most times"	92.8%	94.7%
Staff explained treatment procedures "all" or "most times"	88.9%	82.8%
Staff treated him/her as an individual "all" or "most times"	92.6%	96.2%
Staff respected privacy "all" or "most times"	95.8%	96.5%
Staff available to help "all" or "most times"	94.1%	95.2%
"Would definitely" or "probably" recommend program to friends	98.3%	97.2%

Note. Percentages represent client satisfaction ratings of either "very good" or "excellent."

tions arose, and written instructions for administration were also available.

Analysis Method

To understand which need-vulnerability factors predict client satisfaction (both the single item, four-category assessment and the total sum score index), the Exhaustive CHAID modeling method (Chi-squared Automatic Interaction Detector) is employed (Biggs, de Ville, & Suen, 1991; Huba, 2000; Huba, Panter, & Melchior, 2000). The CHAID modeling approach is quite flexible in its ability to handle different measurement levels for both outcomes (client satisfaction) as well as predictors (need-vulnerability factors). Using an algorithm that searches for optimal associations between the predictors and the outcomes, CHAID sequentially identifies key predictors that most differentiate scores on the outcome variable. Findings from this optimal identification of predictors are assembled in a decision-tree, a graphic that facilitates interpretation of particular client attribute combinations that are most associated with different satisfaction scores. Thus, the total sample of clients is segmented into smaller homogenous groups based on combinations of need-vulnerability factors, which give rise to maximally different client satisfaction scores.

We present two sets of CHAID models. In the first model set we use the 17 need-vulnerability-demographic indicators (from Module 1) to predict the single, four-category client satisfaction rating, and in an alternate model we apply a constraint so that the first predictor variable that is considered is gender. In the second set of models we examine the summed client satisfaction score as the outcome, as predicted by the 17 need-vulnerability-demographic factors. We also check to see whether gender (when constrained to be the first predictor in the model) affects the overall pattern of findings.

Some general model parameters used throughout the analyses are restrictions of the parent node to 10, the child node to 5, and the alpha level for the model tests to .05. For all significance tests, a Bonferroni correction was employed to correct for comparisons made across levels of each predictor included in the CHAID model. We used AnswerTree 2.0 to estimate all models. These analyses were planned and conducted between 1998-2000 by Huba, Melchior, and Panter (1998-2000) for the Knowledge Base on HIV/AIDS Care available at *www.TheMeasurementGroup.com/KB.htm.*

RESULTS

Effects of Predictors on Single-Item, Four-Point Rating of Client Satisfaction

Table 3 shows the individual effects of the predictors on program satisfaction levels using the single-item, four-category rating of overall client satisfaction with services. Three of the 17 possible predictors included here significantly predicted responses on the overall satisfaction rating: age, childcare needs, and illicit drug use (other than crack or heroin). The percentage and number of patients falling into each response category based on these predictors are shown in Table 3.

Model 1 for Client Satisfaction with Services (Single Item)

The first CHAID model, for which the first two splits are shown in Figure 1, uses the dependent measure of the final categorical client satisfaction rating.[3] The predictor variables in the model were the 17 need-vulnerability-demographic factors described above. At the top of the figure, if we consider all 516 individuals, the majority of the clients rated the services received as "very good" or "excellent" (83.7 percent). In the boxes there is a small frequency distribution showing the percentage of clients who fall in each satisfaction category. Because the model relies on empirical rules, the variable in the second row of the tree (from the top) is the predictor that is the "best" way to split the entire sample to differentiate client satisfaction levels. In this model, all splits after the first level are based on statistically significant differences in satisfaction ratings between groups. As shown in the diagram, the optimal split for the sample is by age. Of those 21 years of age or older (the majority of the sample), 83.6 percent rated satisfaction with services as "very good" or "excellent." The 17 individuals under the age of 21 had somewhat less favorable satisfaction ratings, with 58.8 percent of this group rating satisfaction with services as "very good" or "excellent."

For those under 21, the sample was subsequently split on race-ethnicity, although the cell sizes are fairly small at this level. For those participants age 21 or older, the sample was split by childcare needs, substance abuse, and primary language. Based on childcare needs, participants with one child needing care and those with missing data as to childcare needs were relatively less satisfied with these services

TABLE 3. Effects of Need-Vulnerability Factors on Single Item, Four-Category Client Satisfaction Rating

Indicator	Fair/Poor % (n)	Good % (n)	Very Good % (n)	Excellent % (n)	χ^2	df
Age					7.27*	2
Age < 21	17.7 (3)	23.5 (4)	29.4 (5)	29.4 (5)		
Age 21-55	4.3 (21)	11.8 (58)	35.5 (174)	48.4 (237)		
Age > 55	0.0 (0)	33.3 (3)	33.3 (3)	33.3 (3)		
Race-Ethnicity					1.50	3
African American/Black	4.6 (14)	11.8 (36)	38.8 (118)	44.7 (136)		
Hispanic/Latino	5.9 (6)	14.9 (15)	29.7 (30)	49.5 (50)		
Caucasian	3.0 (3)	12.9 (13)	30.7 (31)	53.5 (54)		
Combined Small Groups	10.0 (1)	10.0 (1)	30.0 (3)	50.0 (5)		
Primary Language					2.69	1
English	4.2 (18)	11.3 (48)	36.2 (154)	48.2 (205)		
Not English	6.6 (6)	18.7 (17)	30.8 (28)	44.0 (40)		
Childcare needs					11.70**	3
No Childcare Needs	3.7 (14)	11.0 (42)	36.1 (138)	49.2 (188)		
1 Child Needs Care	8.7 (4)	19.6 (9)	34.8 (16)	37.0 (17)		
> 1 Child Needs Care	0.0 (0)	12.5 (4)	31.3 (10)	56.3 (18)		
Missing	10.7 (6)	17.9 (10)	32.1 (18)	39.3 (22)		
Highest Grade Completed					6.37	3
No HS (< 10)	6.8 (6)	12.5 (11)	37.5 (33)	43.2 (38)		
Some HS (10-11)	4.1 (6)	15.1 (22)	33.6 (49)	47.3 (69)		
HS Grad (12+)	3.2 (6)	8.1 (15)	37.1 (69)	51.6 (96)		
Missing	6.3 (6)	17.7 (17)	32.3 (31)	43.8 (42)		
Employment Status					3.58	3
Employed	4.6 (2)	9.1 (4)	36.4 (16)	50.0 (22)		
Unemployed	4.4 (10)	15.4 (35)	37.9 (86)	42.3 (96)		
Disabled	4.0 (9)	10.2 (23)	35.1 (79)	50.7 (114)		
Missing	15.0 (3)	15.0 (3)	5.0 (1)	65.0 (13)		
Insurance Coverage					3.44	3
Public Insurance	4.9 (11)	10.3 (23)	37.5 (84)	47.3 (106)		
Private Insurance	0.0 (0)	16.7 (5)	20.0 (6)	63.3 (19)		
No Insurance	3.4 (6)	14.3 (25)	36.0 (63)	46.3 (81)		
Missing	8.1 (7)	13.8 (12)	33.3 (29)	44.8 (39)		
Alcohol Problem					6.45	3
No Alcohol Problem	2.7 (2)	12.3 (9)	41.1 (30)	43.8 (32)		
Prior Alcohol Problem	6.9 (9)	13.1 (17)	39.2 (51)	40.8 (53)		
Current Alcohol Problem	4.7 (5)	11.3 (12)	44.3 (47)	39.6 (42)		
Missing	3.9 (8)	13.0 (27)	26.1 (54)	57.0 (118)		
Heroin Use					5.83	3
No Heroin	4.3 (8)	11.4 (21)	44.3 (82)	40.0 (74)		
Prior Heroin	6.7 (7)	14.3 (15)	37.1 (39)	41.9 (44)		
Current Heroin	5.0 (1)	10.0 (2)	35.0 (7)	50.0 (10)		
Missing	3.9 (8)	13.1 (27)	26.2 (54)	56.8 (117)		
Crack Use					6.50	3
No Crack	4.4 (4)	11.1 (10)	37.8 (34)	46.7 (42)		
Prior Crack	4.1 (5)	14.1 (17)	40.5 (49)	41.3 (50)		
Current Crack	7.1 (7)	11.2 (11)	44.9 (44)	36.7 (36)		
Missing	3.9 (8)	13.0 (27)	26.6 (55)	56.5 (117)		

TABLE 3 (continued)

Indicator	Fair/Poor % (n)	Good % (n)	Very Good % (n)	Excellent % (n)	χ^2	df
Other Illicit Drug Use					11.08*	3
No Other Drug	2.7 (3)	10.0 (11)	40.0 (44)	47.3 (52)		
Prior Other Drug	4.7 (7)	14.0 (21)	39.3 (59)	42.0 (63)		
Current Other Drug	12.8 (6)	10.7 (5)	48.9 (23)	27.7 (13)		
Missing	3.8 (8)	13.4 (28)	26.8 (56)	56.0 (117)		
Criminal Justice System (CJS) Involvement					6.90	3
No CJS Involvement	2.9 (3)	8.6 (9)	46.7 (49)	41.9 (44)		
Prior CJS Involvement	8.9 (10)	14.2 (16)	38.1 (43)	38.9 (44)		
Current CJS Involvement	2.3 (2)	10.2 (9)	38.6 (34)	48.9 (43)		
Missing	4.3 (9)	14.8 (31)	26.7 (56)	54.3 (114)		
Sex Work					4.63	3
No Sex Work	2.9 (6)	12.6 (26)	44.0 (91)	40.6 (84)		
Prior Sex Work	5.0 (5)	13.0 (13)	36.0 (36)	46.0 (46)		
Current Sex Work	13.9 (5)	8.3 (3)	36.1 (13)	41.7 (15)		
Missing	4.6 (8)	13.3 (23)	24.3 (42)	57.8 (100)		
Sex with Injection Drug User (IDU)					3.83	3
No Sex with IDU	6.4 (7)	10.9 (12)	38.2 (42)	44.6 (49)		
Prior Sex with IDU	4.1 (5)	18.0 (22)	34.4 (42)	43.4 (53)		
Current Sex with IDU	10.5 (2)	5.3 (1)	47.4 (9)	36.8 (7)		
Missing	3.8 (10)	11.3 (30)	33.6 (89)	51.3 (136)		
Housing Status					0.72	3
Own Home	5.8 (8)	10.8 (15)	33.1 (46)	50.4 (70)		
Friend's Home	4.2 (5)	12.6 (15)	33.6 (40)	49.6 (59)		
Unstable Housing	4.0 (7)	13.2 (23)	40.2 (70)	42.5 (74)		
Missing	4.8 (4)	14.3 (12)	31.0 (26)	50.0 (42)		
Sexual Orientation					5.58	3
Gay/Lesbian	11.6 (5)	18.6 (8)	27.9 (12)	41.9 (18)		
Bisexual	4.6 (1)	18.2 (4)	27.3 (6)	50.0 (11)		
Heterosexual	4.2 (15)	11.9 (43)	38.0 (137)	46.0 (166)		
Unknown	3.3 (3)	11.1 (10)	30.0 (27)	55.6 (50)		
Gender					0.05	1
Male	3.2 (8)	15.2 (38)	33.6 (84)	48.0 (120)		
Female	6.0 (16)	10.2 (27)	36.8 (98)	47.0 (125)		

* $p < .05$, ** $p < .01$, *** $p < .001$
Note. "Prior" denotes the behavior occurred prior to the past 30 days; "Current" denotes the behavior occurred within the past 30 days. The chi-square values shown here are for the relationship of a nominal variable to an ordinal variable (in this case, the overall quality rating) and were calculated using Goodman's (1979) formula in the AnswerTree Program, version 2.1 (SPSS, 1999).

than were patients with no childcare needs or more than one child needing care. Among those with no childcare needs, satisfaction levels were further differentiated by use of illicit drugs other than crack cocaine or heroin. Participants with current drug use, who were former users, or who had missing data as to illicit drug use were satisfied, but less so, than non-users. In the subsample of patients with no childcare needs and missing data regarding other illicit drug use, those

FIGURE 1. First Two Splits in a Fully Empirical Model of a Single-Item Client Satisfaction Rating and Need-Vulnerability-Demographic Factors

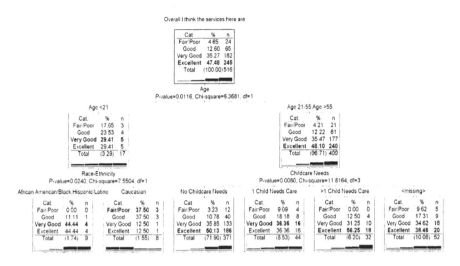

Note. This empirical model shows only statistically significant homogenous groups.

whose primary language was not English were less satisfied than were native English speakers.

Model 2 for Client Satisfaction with Services (Single Item) by Gender

When considering possible CHAID models, the analyst can force a particular ordering of predictor variables, based on theoretical considerations or a desired way to understand client subsamples. The model shown in Figure 2 represents a hybrid CHAID approach that forces gender to be considered as the first predictor in the model, followed by an empirical consideration and optimal identification of the other 16 possible predictors for the model. Figure 2 shows the first two splits in this model. Of the 250 males, 81.6 percent rated services received as "very good" or "excellent," whereas 83.8 percent of the 266 females rated services received as "very good" or "excellent." It should be noted that there was no statistically significant gender difference in ratings of satisfaction with services ($p > .05$), and hence Model 1 is more parsimonious, although this model serves to illustrate gender-specific findings. Among satisfaction scores, females were further

FIGURE 2. First Two Splits in a Model of a Single-Item Client Satisfaction Rating and Need-Vulnerability-Demographic Factors: Gender at First Split with Subsequent Empirical Model

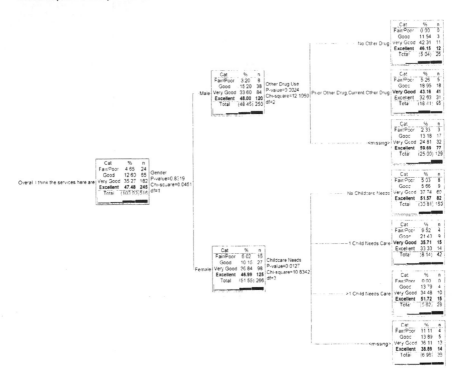

Note. The model was empirically derived after the first split on gender. After the initial gender split, only statistically significant groupings are included in the model.

differentiated based on childcare needs. As in Model 1, female patients with one child needing care and those with missing data as to childcare needs rated their satisfaction with HIV/AIDS services lower than did females with no childcare needs or more than one child needing care. On the other hand, satisfaction levels among male HIV/AIDS patients were first differentiated by illicit drug use (other than crack cocaine or heroin). Participants with a prior or current history of drug use were less satisfied than were those with no other illicit drug use or missing data on that indicator. Among the male HIV/AIDS patients with missing data for drug use, satisfaction levels were further split based on primary language, with non-native English speakers less satisfied. Finally, those with English as their primary language were further differentiated by sexual orientation. Although the number of respondents in each category is relatively small at the bottom of the model, gay/bisexual males whose primary language is English and with an unknown history of illicit drug use tend to have the lowest levels of client satisfaction.

Effects of Predictors on Total Patient Satisfaction Scores

As an alternative to using the overall satisfaction item response as the dependent measure, we also examined whether gender and the need-vulnerability indicators predicted the sum score of client satisfaction. Recall that total satisfaction scores could range from 8 ("least satisfied") to 32 ("most satisfied"). For the following analyses, individual response items were summed to produce a total satisfaction score for each client. Table 4 shows how the individual needs predict total client satisfaction scores. Three of the 17 possible predictors showed significant mean differences on total satisfaction score: age, childcare needs, and sexual orientation. The mean and standard deviation for the total satisfaction score, as well as the number of persons in each group based on the predictors are shown in Table 4.

Model 1 for Total Client Satisfaction with Program (Total Score)

Figure 3 shows the first two splits in a purely empirical model fit to total client satisfaction ratings. Note that this figure looks slightly different than Figures 1 and 2 because the dependent variable is now a quantitative (continuous) variable (total client satisfaction score) rather than a categorical one (single item, four-point client satisfaction rating). The individual boxes show the distribution of the patients at that node on the total satisfaction score. In all cases, as expected, satisfaction scores are very high. Among all 516 clients in this sample, the mean satisfaction score was 28.86. The first optimal split on client satisfaction for the sample was based on age. On average, the most satisfied participants were the 499 clients who were 21 years of age or older (mean satisfaction = 29.02). The group under 21 years of age reported a mean satisfaction score of 24.35 ($p < .0001$). The group of eight persons who were under the age of 21 years and Caucasian, as can be seen in Figure 3, were the least satisfied group in these analyses (mean satisfaction = 19.38).

TABLE 4. Effects of Need-Vulnerability Factors on Total Client Satisfaction Score

Indicator	M	SD	n	%	F	df
Age					12.63***	2, 513
Age < 21	24.35	7.17	17	3.3		
Age 21-55	29.03	3.61	490	95.0		
Age > 55	28.56	3.57	9	1.7		
Race-Ethnicity					0.58	3, 512
African American/Black	28.96	3.51	304	58.9		
Hispanic/Latino	28.42	4.34	101	19.6		
Caucasian	28.99	4.41	101	19.6		
Combined Small Groups	29.20	2.94	10	1.9		
Language not English					0.14	1, 514
English	28.89	3.81	425	82.4		
Not English	28.73	4.09	91	17.6		
Childcare needs					4.31**	3, 512
No Childcare Needs	29.09	3.59	382	74.0		
1 Child Needs Care	27.72	4.93	46	8.9		
> 1 Child Needs Care	29.87	2.98	32	6.2		
Missing	27.69	4.66	56	10.9		
Highest Grade Completed					0.39	3, 512
No HS (< Grade 10)	28.91	3.93	88	17.1		
Some HS (Grade 10-11)	28.64	3.80	146	28.3		
HS grad (Grade 12+ or GED)	29.08	3.88	186	36.1		
Missing	28.74	3.88	96	18.6		
Employment Status					0.86	3, 512
Employed	28.84	3.25	44	8.5		
Unemployed	28.60	4.27	227	44.0		
Disabled	29.16	3.36	225	43.6		
Missing	28.50	5.32	20	3.8		
Insurance Coverage					0.50	3, 512
Public Insurance	29.00	3.72	224	43.4		
Private Insurance	29.43	3.61	30	5.8		
No Insurance	28.66	4.01	175	34.0		
Missing	28.75	4.00	87	16.9		
Alcohol Problem					2.23	3, 512
No Alcohol Problem	28.74	3.79	73	14.2		
Prior Alcohol Problem	28.44	4.28	130	25.2		
Current Alcohol Problem	28.45	3.47	106	20.5		
Missing	29.39	3.75	207	40.1		
Heroin Use					1.71	3, 512
No Heroin	28.50	3.85	185	35.9		
Prior Heroin	28.66	3.94	105	20.4		
Current Heroin	28.55	4.41	20	3.9		
Missing	29.33	3.75	206	39.9		
Crack Use					2.28	3, 512
No Crack	28.90	3.73	110	21.3		
Prior Crack	28.47	4.08	121	23.5		
Current Crack	28.29	3.86	98	19.0		
Missing	29.35	3.75	207	40.1		
Other Illicit Drug Use					2.29	3, 512
No Other Drug	29.00	3.69	110	21.3		
Prior Other Drug	28.59	3.86	150	29.1		
Current Other Drug	27.74	4.06	9.1	27.7		
Missing	29.24	3.86	209	40.5		

TABLE 4 (continued)

Indicator	M	SD	n	%	F	df
Criminal Justice System (CJS) Involved					2.58	3, 512
No CJS Involvement	28.96	3.31	105	20.4		
Prior CJS Involvement	28.00	4.39	113	22.0		
Current CJS Involvement	29.32	3.23	88	17.1		
Missing	29.09	4.00	210	40.7		
Sex Work					1.34	3, 512
No Sex Work	28.85	3.30	207	40.1		
Prior Sex Work	28.65	4.25	100	19.4		
Current Sex Work	27.86	5.09	36	7.0		
Missing	29.20	3.94	173	33.5		
Sex with Injection Drug User (IDU)					0.77	3, 512
No Sex with IDU	28.73	4.00	110	21.3		
Prior Sex with IDU	28.70	3.93	122	23.6		
Current Sex with IDU	27.89	4.78	19	3.7		
Missing	29.10	3.69	265	51.3		
Housing Status					1.08	3, 512
Own Home	29.22	3.24	139	26.9		
Friend's Home	28.87	3.98	119	23.1		
Unstable Housing	28.47	4.40	174	33.7		
Missing	29.08	3.40	84	16.3		
Sexual Orientation					4.52**	3, 512
Gay/Lesbian	27.19	5.96	43	8.3		
Bisexual	27.36	5.43	22	4.3		
Heterosexual	29.06	3.38	361	70.0		
Unknown	29.24	3.71	90	17.4		
Gender					0.03	1, 514
Male	28.84	4.03	250	48.5		
Female	28.89	3.69	266	51.6		

$* p < .05, ** p < .01, *** p < .001$

Note. "Prior" denotes the behavior occurred prior to the past 30 days; "Current" denotes the behavior occurred within the past 30 days.

Among respondents over 21 years of age, the pattern of total satisfaction scores was similar to that obtained when predicting levels on the single satisfaction rating in Models 1 and 2. In this case, total satisfaction scores were first split by childcare needs, followed by other illicit drug use, gender, and primary language. Female HIV/AIDS patients who were drug users with no child care needs had higher total satisfaction scores (mean satisfaction = 29.16) than did male HIV/AIDS patients with the same characteristics (mean satisfaction = 27.96). Finally, the females were split again based on problem alcohol use. Women with prior alcohol problems (mean satisfaction = 30.32) were more satisfied on average than were females in this group with no alcohol problem (mean satisfaction = 28.75) or a current alcohol problem (mean satisfaction = 28.09).

FIGURE 3. First Two Splits in a Fully Empirical Model of Total Client Satisfaction Scores and Need-Vulnerability-Demographic Factors

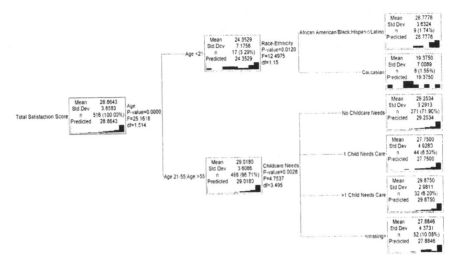

Note. This empirical model is based on the total for eight client satisfaction items. Total scores were determined by summing client ratings for eight items. Each item could be rated from "least satisfied" (1) to "most satisfied" (4).

Model 2 for Total Client Satisfaction with Program (Total Score) by Gender

As an alternative to the model shown in Figure 3 for the total client satisfaction ratings, we also developed a model for the same data in which the split at the first level was forced to be gender. The mean client satisfaction scores between genders were not statistically different, and again, the prior presented model may be considered to be more parsimonious. Satisfaction with services ratings for males and females were 28.84 and 28.89, respectively. Following the forced split on gender, the data were split empirically. Among males, the sample split on age, illicit drug use (other than crack cocaine or heroin), and sexual orientation. The first two splits in this model are given in Figure 4. As in earlier analyses, males under the age of 21 reported significantly less satisfaction with services (mean satisfaction = 22.73) than males who were 21 years or older (mean satisfaction = 29.12). Drug use, either prior or current, predicted lower satisfaction scores for males 21 years of age or older. For males with missing data as to illicit drug use, being gay or bisexual predicted slightly lower mean

FIGURE 4. First Two Splits in a Model of Client Satisfaction Scores and Need-Vulnerability-Demographic Factors: Gender at First Split with Subsequent Empirical Model

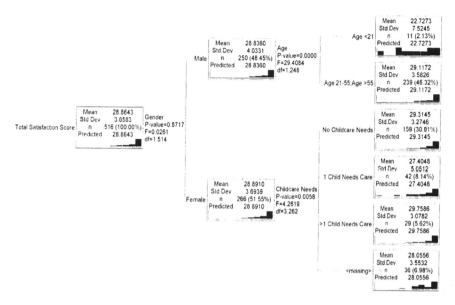

Note. The first gender split in this model was forced. All subsequent groupings were derived empirically. The score is based on the sum of ratings on eight client satisfaction items.

satisfaction scores, although the number of individuals in those groups is quite small. Among females, satisfaction levels were differentiated by childcare needs and sexual orientation. Women who did not have childcare needs or who had more than one child needing care reported slightly higher satisfaction levels. Females with no childcare needs and bisexual or unknown orientation were least satisfied. The sample sizes for lesbian and bisexual females with no childcare needs are quite small and must be interpreted with caution.

DISCUSSION

In this article, a method for splitting a sample based on a large number of possible predictors (Huba, Panter, & Melchior, 2000) was used to study client satisfaction with services in seven innovative models of HIV/AIDS care. The results indicate that satisfaction was extremely high in all program participant groups. Differences in the level of satisfaction vary slightly, and only small groups of clients report somewhat lower satisfaction scores than the overall study population.

Predicting satisfaction levels using two different indicators yielded similar, but not identical models. This finding suggests that examining overall levels of satisfaction, as well as response patterns within different patient groups may yield different types of information. Use of multiple modeling strategies, indicator types, and data sources can better illustrate the ways that satisfaction with care may differ among various treatment populations.

These results highlight that focusing on the cultural, social and behavioral attributes of specific groups in designing and implementing service and treatment programs for HIV/AIDS patients has a positive and profound impact on client satisfaction. Overall client satisfaction with services was rated very highly. Satisfaction scores, both the single item, four-category index and the summed client satisfaction score, did not vary significantly among the majority of socio-demographic and behavioral categories.

As expected, based on prior research, lower ratings of client satisfaction with services came from males under the age of 21. Indicators of needing childcare and/or speaking a language other than English also predicted lower satisfaction scores. Similar findings regarding decreased satisfaction with services for these groups in treatment were reported by Knowlton, Latkin, Celentano and Hoover (1998).

The overall high degree of client satisfaction reported for the six CBOs and one comprehensive healthcare clinic in this study is, in part, based on higher levels of satisfaction with services reported by groups of persons of color and women. Recent reports on client satisfaction for these groups shows that women and minorities often experience higher levels of *dis*satisfaction with treatment than any other groups and report greater barriers in access to treatments (Rapkin et al., 1998; Eversley, Israelski, Smith, & Kunwar, 1998). In the Eversley et al. study, their sample of women of color recorded a greater level of dissatisfaction with services compared to Caucasian counterparts. In the present study sample, however, people of color reported extremely high levels of satisfaction with services.

The difference in findings in the present study can partially be explained by the approach taken by the projects highlighted in this investigation. Each project utilized a program design and implementation methodology that explicitly included aligning their services with client needs. In addition, these providers constructed service delivery systems that were culturally and socially appropriate to fit the characteristics of their clients. Third, these programs were committed to continuously monitoring client satisfaction. Client satisfaction data were gathered on a routine basis from clients from their entry into the programs. Continuous monitoring of client satisfaction as a routine part of service delivery assures program leadership and staff that client feedback about services is an important part of how the organization assures that its clients receive quality and effective services.

The CHAID analysis utilized in reporting the results in this article also has significant potential for the future development and operations of HIV programs interested in constructing an effective client monitoring system. While the technical aspects of this analytical tool may be beyond the capabilities of some CBOs, the methods used in the CHAID process for aggregating client data by clinically, socially and culturally meaningful cohorts has profound implications for a CBO's ability to comprehend the service segments within its client base. The CBOs and university clinic in this study, through the analysis of client satisfaction data, which permitted client sub-groupings and sub-group comparisons, were given the ability to understand how their service programming and implementation impacted each of these groups. This sophisticated market segmentation approach (Huba, Panter, & Melchior, 2000) to understanding service delivery permits service organizations to focus improvements, to provide enhancements to services, and to make appropriate service changes. These changes can be targeted at maximum points of leverage with the overall program service delivery system. HIV service providers to potentially difficult, problematic and heterogeneous client groups should adapt a strategy of segmenting the monitoring and analysis of client feedback data to be able to work on clients' needs in a focused and meaningful way.

AUTHOR NOTES

This study was supported in part by Health Resources and Services Administration (HRSA), HIV/AIDS Bureau (HAB), Special Projects of National Significance (SPNS) Grant Number 5 U90 HA 00030-05 for the work of the Evaluation and Dissemination Center and by grants to the individual projects. This article's contents are solely the responsibility of the authors and do not necessarily represent the official view of the funding agency. From PROTOTYPES (V. Brown), from The Measurement Group (L. Melchior, G. Huba), from The Fortune Society (T. Gallagher), from the Center for Community Health Education and Research (E. Jean-Louis, J. Walker), from Outreach, Inc. (S. McDonald), from the University of Vermont School of Medicine (K. Richardson-Nassif), from the Well-Being Institute (G. Smereck), from Larkin Street Youth Center (A. Stanton), from the Health Resources and Services Administration (K. Marconi), from the University of North Carolina, Chapel Hill and The Measurement Group (A. Panter), and from the University of Washington, School of Social Work and the Visiting Nurse Association Foundation (D. Cherin). The analyses for this paper were planned and conducted between 1998-2000 by Huba, Melchior, and Panter (1998-2000) for the Knowledge Base on HIV/AIDS Care available at *www.TheMeasurementGroup.com/KB.htm*. Special thanks to Rupinder K. Sidhu, Cindy T. Le, Chermeen Elavia, and Kimberly Ishihara for help with manuscript preparation, to Jocelyn Medina and Katherine Ellingson for help with data processing, and to the late Diana E. Brief, PhD, for help with data management, all of The Measurement Group.

NOTES

1. Human Subject Protection Committee at each site determined if informed consent for participation in the evaluation was required, or if the data were collected as part of the usual quality improvement process, and hence exempt. All data collection at all sites was voluntary for clients and providers, and hence, these data do have certain non-random patterns of missing observations.

2. If there were fewer than four items with missing data on the client satisfaction scale, values were imputed using the EM algorithm.

3. Because of space limitations due to printing at this size, the models shown in Figures 1 through 4 are limited to three levels (two splits) each. Supplemental figures showing the complete models in full color are available online at *www.TheMeasurement Group.com/HHC/clientsatis.htm*.

REFERENCES

Aiken, L., Sloane, D., Lake, E., Sochalski, J., & Weber, A. (1999). Organization and outcomes of inpatient AIDS care. *Medical Care, 37* (8), 760-772.

Biggs, D., de Ville, B., & Suen, E. (1991). A method of choosing multiway partitions for classification and decision trees. *Journal of Applied Statistics, 18*, 49-62.

Brown, V. B., Stanton, A., Smereck, G., McDonald, S., Gallagher, T., Jean-Louis, E., Hughes, C., Kemp, J. W., Kennedy, M., & Brief, D. E. (2000). Lessons learned in reducing barriers to care: Reflections from the community perspective. *Drugs & Society, 16*(1/2), 55-74.

Burke, J., Cohen, J., Weber, K., Garcia, P., Sha, B., & Hershow, R. (1998). Sources of dissatisfaction with health care among HIV+ women in the women's interagency HIV study. *International Conference on AIDS, 12*, 101. (Abstract No. 12442).

Centers for Disease Control and Prevention (1999). *HIV/AIDS Surveillance Report*, *11* (1), 1-44.

Eversley, R., Israelski, D., Smith, S., & Kunwar, P. (1998). Satisfaction with medical care associated with race, HIV symptoms and recovery from substance abuse among HIV-infected women. *International Conference on AIDS*, *12*, 815-6. (Abstract No. 42214).

Huba, G. J. (2001). Introduction: Evaluating HIV/AIDS treatment programs for underserved and vulnerable patients, innovative methods and findings. *Home Health Care Services Quarterly: The Journal of Community Care, 19*(1/2), 1-6.

Huba, G. J., Brown, V. B., Melchior, L. A., Hughes, C., & Panter, A. T. (2000). Conceptual issues in implementing and using evaluation in the "real world" setting of a community-based organization for HIV/AIDS services. *Drugs & Society, 16*(1/2), 31-54.

Huba, G. J., Melchior, L. A., & Panter, A. T. (1998-2000). Knowledge Base on HIV/AIDS Care. Online: *www.TheMeasurementGroup.com/KB.htm.*

Huba, G. J., Melchior, L. A., Brown, V. B., Larson, T. A., & Panter, A. T. (Eds.). (2000). Evaluating HIV/AIDS Treatment Programs: Innovative Methods and Findings [Special Issue]. *Drugs & Society, 16*(1/2).

Huba, G. J., Melchior, L. A., De Veauuse, N., Hillary, K., Singer, B., & Marconi, K. (1998). A national program of AIDS capitated care projects and their evaluation. *Home Health Care Services Quarterly, 17 (1)*, 3-30.

Huba, G. J., Melchior, L. A., Panter, A. T., Brown, V. B., & Larson, T. L. (2000). A national program of AIDS care projects and their cross-cutting evaluation: The HRSA SPNS Cooperative Agreements. *Drugs & Society, 16*(1/2), 5-29.

Huba, G. J., Melchior, L. A., Panter, A. T., Smereck, G., Meredith, K., Cherin, D. A., Richardson-Nassif, K., German, V. F., Rohweder, C., Brown, V. B., McDonald, S., Kaplan, J., Stanton, A., Chase, P., Jean-Louis, E., Gallagher, T., Steinberg, J., Reis, P., Mundy, L., & Larson, T. A. (2000). Psychometric scaling of a disenfranchisement index for HIV service need. Manuscript in preparation.

Huba, G. J., Melchior, L. A., Staff of The Measurement Group, & the HRSA SPNS Cooperative Agreement Projects. (1997a). *Module 1: Demographics-Contact Form.* Online: *www.TheMeasurementGroup.com/modules.htm.*

Huba, G. J., Melchior, L. A., Staff of The Measurement Group, & the HRSA SPNS Cooperative Agreement Projects. (1997b). *Module 11: Client Satisfaction Survey.* Online: *www.TheMeasurementGroup.com/modules.htm.*

Huba, G. J., Panter, A. T., & Melchior, L. A. (2000). Empirical modeling of patient characteristics and services using sample partitioning, interaction detection, or classification tree methods: Practical issues and recommendations. Manuscript in preparation.

Johnson, L. M. (1994). An assessment of satisfaction of clinical research participants in a long-term care study. *International Conference on AIDS*, *10* (2), 393. (Abstract No. 755).

Knowlton, A., Latkin, C. A., Celentano, D. D., & Hoover, D. R. (1998). Predictors of satisfaction with informal caregivers among lower class injection drug users affected by HIV. *International Conference on AIDS*, *12*, 473. (Abstract No. 24163).

Lucas, J. (1999). High active antiretroviral therapy in a large urban clinic: Risk factors. *Annals of Internal Medicine, 131* (2), 81-7.

Morrow, K. M., & Fuqua, R. W. (1997). Women who have sex with women: Consumer satisfaction with an HIV/STD prevention program. *National Conference on Women and HIV,* 166. (Abstract No. P1.44).

Patti, R. (1987). Managing for service effectiveness in social welfare: Toward a performance model. *Administration in Social Work, 11,* (3-4), 7-22.

Poertner, J. (1986). The use of client feedback to improve practice. *The Clinical Supervisor, 4* (4), 57-66.

Pounds, M., Finkelstein, E., Warfield, P., & Park, J. C. (1998). Client satisfaction activities and Ryan White Care Act: Involving people living with HIV and improving systems of care. *International Conference on AIDS, 12,* 103. (Abstract No. 12451).

Powell-Cope, G. M., Brown, M. A., Holzemer, W. L., Corless, I. B., Turner, J. G., Nokes, K. M., & Inouye, J. (1998). Perceived health care providers support and HIV adherence. *International Conference on AIDS, 12,* 592. (Abstract No. 32354).

Rapkin, B., Smith, M., Feldman, I., Cruz, H., Plavin, H., & Jemiolo, D. (1998). Access and barriers to care among HIV+ Medicaid recipients. *International Conference on AIDS, 12,* 833-4. (Abstract No. 42301).

Rapp, C., & Poertner, J. (1987). Moving clients center stage through the use of client outcomes. In Patti, R., Poertner, J., & Rapp, C. (Eds.). *Managing for service effectiveness in social welfare organizations.* New York: The Haworth Press, Inc.

Rapp, C., & Poertner, J. (1992). *Social administration: A client-centered approach.* New York: Longman.

Richardson-Nassif, K., Meredith, K. L., Larson, T. A., Mundy, L. M., & Melchior, L. A. (in press). Integrating and utilizing evaluation in comprehensive HIV care programs. *Drugs & Society.*

Scott-Lennox, J., Braun, J. F., Morrow, J. E., Lawson, K., Tirelli, R., Dietrich, D., Hergenroeder, P., Kreiswirth, S., McMeeking, A., Mullen, M., & Weiz, K. (1998). Development of the HIV Treatment Satisfaction Survey (HTSS) to improve adherence and quality. *International Conference on AIDS, 12,* 102. (Abstract No. 12445).

SPSS. (1999). *AnswerTree,* version 2.1 (computer software).

Satisfaction with Services in Innovative Managed Care Programs for Groups of Traditionally Underserved Individuals with HIV/AIDS: Empirical Models

David A. Cherin, PhD
G. J. Huba, PhD
Judith Steinberg, MD
Peter Reis
Lisa A. Melchior, PhD
Katherine Marconi, PhD
A. T. Panter, PhD

SUMMARY. As the number of people with HIV/AIDS receiving services in managed care models increases, concerns over quality of care and satisfaction with services have grown. This article examined data from three national demonstration projects that were funded to enroll traditionally underserved individuals and provide innovative medical services in programs developing models appropriate for managed care funding. Assessments of patient satisfaction were related to indicators of traditionally underserved status including demographic characteristics, behaviors, and other risk factors using the data modeling method of Exhaustive CHAID (Chi-squared Automatic Interaction Detector).

Address correspondence to: G. J. Huba, PhD, The Measurement Group, 5811A Uplander Way, Culver City, CA 90230 (E-mail: *ghuba@TheMeasurementGroup. com*).

[Haworth co-indexing entry note]: "Satisfaction with Services in Innovative Managed Care Programs for Groups of Traditionally Underserved Individuals with HIV/AIDS: Empirical Models." Cherin, David A. et al. Co-published simultaneously in *Home Health Care Services Quarterly* (The Haworth Press, Inc.) Vol. 19, No. 1/2, 2001, pp. 103-125; and: *The Next Generation of AIDS Patients: Service Needs and Vulnerabilities* (ed: George J. Huba et al.) The Haworth Press, Inc., 2001, pp. 103-125. Single or multiple copies of this article are available for a fee from The Haworth Document Delivery Service [1-800-342-9678, 9:00 a.m. - 5:00 p.m. (EST). E-mail address: getinfo@haworthpressinc.com].

Overall patient satisfaction levels with these programs were very high. Through the modeling methods, the groups most likely to experience the greatest program satisfaction are identified. In general, all groups were highly satisfied with the programs. *[Article copies available for a fee from The Haworth Document Delivery Service: 1-800-342-9678. E-mail address: <getinfo@haworthpressinc.com> Website: <http://www.HaworthPress. com> © 2001 by The Haworth Press, Inc. All rights reserved.]*

KEYWORDS. HIV/AIDS, patient satisfaction, underserved, CHAID

As states across the United States move toward enrollment of their Medicaid populations into managed care arrangements, HIV/AIDS patients are at considerable risk for encountering quality of care problems and barriers to accessing care. Given the complex nature of HIV/AIDS, the moves by states to reduce the cost of care can also produce unexpected barriers to treatment. This critical issue requires continuous monitoring of quality of care and patient satisfaction with care by providers, payers, and funders working with and on behalf of HIV populations and HIV/AIDS patients themselves.

Pressure to reduce health care costs in the U.S. has led to dramatic increases in patient enrollment with managed care organizations. . . The growth in managed care has primarily involved increasing enrollment of healthy, employed individuals, while these populations may benefit from reduction in unnecessary care, individuals with resource intensive chronic illnesses such as HIV may be at risk for under-treatment. (Kitahata, Holmes, Wagner, & Gooding, 1998, p. 511)

Patient satisfaction with services, as a cornerstone of quality care, has emerged as an important focus of managed care organizations (MCOs) over the last decade. Member dissatisfaction with services has been demonstrated to have a direct impact on plan disenrollment (Weiss & Senf, 1990). Katz and colleagues (Katz, Marx, Douglas, Bolan, Park, Gurley, & Buchbinder, 1997) note that patient satisfaction is a valuable indicator of the quality of medical care and is an extremely important measure for medical plans serving HIV/AIDS patients. "Evaluating satisfaction with medical care among HIV-infected persons is important because satisfaction has been shown to be associated with. . . adherence to medical treatment" (p. 2). Given the vulnerable nature of HIV/AIDS patients and the complexity of conditions with which they must live, disenrolling from their health plans can have a profound negative impact on the continuity of their treatments, the costs of care, and ultimately, the outcomes of care. Current HIV/AIDS patients, who have historically reported difficulties with access to mainstream care, are extremely vulnerable to disrupted treatment if their satisfaction with care is not considered by managed care providers in designing and implementing services. The combination of these medical, social, and cultural dynamics require that managed care organizations treating HIV/AIDS patients continuously monitor patient satisfaction with services as a primary strategy to insure quality of care and work toward positive treatment outcomes.

PATIENT SATISFACTION AND MANAGED CARE

A number of leading health and managed care industry research institutions have spent a considerable amount of time in the last decade building and refining patient satisfaction with services instruments tailored to MCOs. Among those groups are the Group Health Association of America (GHAA), the RAND Corporation, and The Measurement Group (TMG). GHAA is the professional trade organization that represents the managed care industry, and RAND is a large research and policy based organization. Both have developed medical patient satisfaction questionnaires tailored for managed care settings, the Consumer Satisfaction Survey and the MOS, respectively. The MOS has been adapted by RAND to be used with MCOs. The Measurement Group has, in its work with the Health Resources and Services Administration HIV/AIDS Bureau, developed and tested a patient satisfaction questionnaire that was specifically designed for HIV/AIDS patients in managed care plans.

In general, these instruments define satisfaction in the managed care context as a patient's perceived quality of program physicians, access to services, communications with providers and with administrative staff, and perceptions of the success of stated outcomes of treatment (Wilson, Sullivan, & Weissman, 1998; Huba, Melchior, Staff of The Measurement Group, & the HRSA SPNS Cooperative Agreement Projects, 1997b; Jatulis, Bundek, & Legorreta, 1997). Specifically, the focus on patient satisfaction revolves around the domains of the patient's: (1) perceived technical capabilities and disease specific expertise of both physicians and nurses; (2) views of the interpersonal relationships with staff; (3) experiences with accessing providers, especially after clinic business hours; (4) perceptions of the communications with providers as well as program staff; (5) perceptions of time spent with them by providers in answering questions and providing important treatment information; and (6) perceptions of the outcomes of treatment.

Patient satisfaction with services in a managed care environment is a multidimensional concept linked inextricably to the technical expertise of care providers, the ability of the managed care organizations to ensure access to care, and the provision of a seamless continuum of services. In addition, managed care providers must focus on these factors while also managing the costs of care and the risks associated with treating a resource intensive illness like HIV/AIDS. Patient satisfaction, therefore, is at the critical intersection between how patients perceive their encounters with direct care providers and how they perceive their encounters with the managed care institution.

To balance the two dimensions of patient satisfaction, HIV/AIDS managed care providers need to understand that cost of care and comprehensiveness of care are not mutually exclusive. Managed care providers serving HIV/AIDS patients should view capitated reimbursement and the need to deliver a full range of accessible services as complimentary incentives to deliver care and to provide services as effectively as possible. To maximize patient satisfaction under these conditions, managed care organizations need to develop sound protocols for: (1) coordinating care and case management; (2) assuring the HIV/AIDS expertise of their primary physicians and creating a system of knowledge keepers; (3) engaging patients in the design and implementing services; (4) providing ongoing education to patient and staff; and (5) developing information systems that will provide evidence-based costs of care and treatment (Kitahata et al., 1998; Powell, O'Neill, Holloway, & Gomez, 1998; Katz et al., 1997). These guidelines were incorporated into the design and implementation of the managed care programs described in this article.

THREE INNOVATIVE MANAGED CARE PROVIDERS

In 1994, the HIV/AIDS Bureau of the Health Resources and Services Administration (HRSA) funded Special Projects of National Significance (SPNS) to develop innovative HIV/AIDS service models. Three projects, conducted by the Johns Hopkins University Moore Clinic (Baltimore, Maryland), East Boston Neighborhood Health Center (East Boston, Massachusetts), and AIDS Healthcare Foundation (Los Angeles, California), focused on medical or medical support services provided in clinics developing innovative models for a managed care environment. The three projects are located throughout the United States, focus on somewhat different target populations, and use somewhat different strategies for recruiting and treating patients. Overall, however, each program has tried to address the issues of finding individuals who have not had full access to state-of-the-art medical services and then providing appropriate treatment. Table 1 gives a brief description of the three projects and their strategies for recruiting hard-to-reach populations and delivering services. Each of the three providers offered their patients the full continuum of acute and community-based services within a managed care environment. Each program developed models of care that fully preserved HIV specialty services in the community and took the approach of developing capitation rates based on patient needs that accurately reflected the intensity of required services. Additional information about these managed care service models is available at *www.TheMeasurement Group.com/KB.htm* (Huba, Melchior, & Panter, 1998-2000).

METHOD

Participants

The 384 patients in this sample received services at one of three of the national demonstration projects funded as HRSA HIV/AIDS Bureau Special Projects of National Significance (SPNS). All of the participants were HIV-positive. Of the 257 males, 51.4 percent were African American, 18.3 percent were Hispanic/Latino, 29.2 percent were Caucasian, and 1.2 percent were Asian-Pacific Islander. Of the 127 females, 73.2 percent were African American, 8.7 percent were Hispanic/Latina, and 18.1 percent were Caucasian.

Instruments and Indicators

As part of their involvement in the cooperative agreement, projects agreed to participate in a cross-cutting evaluation (see Huba, Mel-

TABLE 1. Three SPNS Cooperative Agreement Projects: Project Summaries

Project	Grant Title	Description
AIDS Healthcare Foundation (Los Angeles, California)	Test the Feasibility of Providing Comprehensive HIV Services Under a Capitated Reimbursement System	AIDS Healthcare Foundation is demonstrating that an enhanced, capitated, managed health care approach to providing HIV/AIDS care will produce fewer opportunistic infections, fewer and shorter hospitalizations, better compliance with medical treatment, and an overall longer life span, including a better quality of life for HIV/AIDS diagnosed populations.
East Boston Neighborhood Health Center (East Boston, Massachusetts)	Development of an HIV/AIDS Service Delivery Model	By exploring the feasibility of developing three separate, capitated reimbursement rates for patients who will be appropriately grouped according to clinical diagnosis–HIV-positive asymptomatic, HIV-positive symptomatic, and CDC AIDS–the East Boston Neighborhood Health Center is developing a cost-efficient, community-based HIV/AIDS care plan.
Johns Hopkins University School of Medicine (Baltimore, Maryland)	Johns Hopkins–Medicaid AIDS Capitated Care Program	The Johns Hopkins University School of Medicine is reducing the financial barriers to adequate care for AIDS patients and to improve the comprehensiveness of their care, while containing costs to the insurer and reducing uncompensated costs to the provider.

chior, De Veauuse, Hillary, Singer, & Marconi, 1998; Huba, Melchior, Panter, Brown, & Larson, 2000). The cross-cutting evaluation included standardized forms used to track activities of individual participants. Sociodemographic data were collected using *Module 1: Demographics-Contact Form* (Huba, Melchior, Staff of The Measurement Group, & the HRSA SPNS Cooperative Agreement Projects, 1997a). Data pertaining to patient satisfaction were gathered with the *Module 11: Patient Satisfaction Survey* (Huba, Melchior, Staff of The Measurement Group, & the HRSA SPNS Cooperative Agreement Projects, 1997b). Interview protocols are presented at *www.TheMeasurement Group.com/Modules.htm.*

Background characteristics. Module 1 was used to document participant characteristics at program enrollment and to update information periodically as new facts about the individual became available. In the cases where multiple Module 1 forms were available for a participant, the greatest level of risk across forms was coded. In addition to demographic characteristics such as gender, age, and ethnicity, a number of behaviors were coded indicating various factors associated with risk for HIV infection and transmission, as well as other measures of need among the HIV patients. A related investigation (Huba, Melchior, Panter, Smereck, Meredith, Cherin, Richardson-Nassif, German, Rohweder, Brown, McDonald, Kaplan, Stanton, Chase, Jean-Louis, Gallagher, Steinberg, Reis, Mundy, & Larson, 2000) developed an index of need for HIV/AIDS patients served by these service demonstration programs.

Predictors. From the information collected on Module 1, a set of 17 indicators was coded to reflect service needs, vulnerabilities, and demographic characteristics. These variables included Gender (Male, Female); Sexual Orientation (Gay/Lesbian, Bisexual, Heterosexual, Unknown); Age (Less than 21, 21-55, Over 55); Race-Ethnicity (African American/Black, Hispanic/Latino, Caucasian, Combined Small Groups); Primary Language (English, Not English); Childcare Needs (No Childcare Needs, One Child Needs Care, More than One Child Needs Care); Highest Grade Completed (No High School–< 10, Some High School–10-11, High School Grad–12+); Employment Status (Employed, Unemployed, Disabled); Insurance Coverage (Public Insurance, Private Insurance, No Insurance); Problem Alcohol Use (No Alcohol Problem, Prior Alcohol Problem, Current Alcohol Problem); Heroin Use (No Heroin, Prior Heroin, Current Heroin); Crack Cocaine

Use (No Crack, Prior Crack, Current Crack); Other Illicit Drug Use (No Other Drug, Prior Other Drug, Current Other Drug); Involvement with the Criminal Justice System (CJS; No CJS, Prior CJS, Current CJS); Sex Work (No Sex Work, Prior Sex Work, Current Sex Work); Sex with an Injection Drug User (IDU; No Sex with IDU, Prior Sex with IDU, Current Sex with IDU); and Housing Status (Own Home, Friend's Home, Unstable Housing). Indicators coded as "current" indicated the risk occurred within 30 days of the assessment, while those coded as "prior" indicated the risk occurred prior to 30 days before assessment, with the most severe level of risk noted during the service episode. Further detail about the derivation of these indicators is available online at *www.TheMeasurementGroup.com/KB.htm* (Huba, Melchior, & Panter, 1998-2000).

Patient satisfaction indicators. Patient satisfaction data were collected using *Module 11: Patient Satisfaction Survey* (Huba, Melchior, Staff of The Measurement Group, & the HRSA SPNS Cooperative Agreement Projects, 1997b). Module 11 was used to document ratings of patient satisfaction with services and the overall program.

For these analyses, we used two different indices of satisfaction with services. The first index was the single item, categorical rating of overall satisfaction with services. This item was coded as fair/poor, good, very good, or excellent.

The second index used to denote patient satisfaction was the sum of all satisfaction items. This sum includes the categorical rating index, as well as eight other indicators of patient satisfaction. Thus, the sum score of patient satisfaction is more reliable and includes the single item index. The range of this satisfaction score is 9 to 36. Satisfaction ratings were selected for analysis if they were the last satisfaction assessments obtained from the participant. These "final" satisfaction ratings were obtained an average of 403.49 days (s.d. = 344.78 days) from program enrollment, with a range of 61 to 1651 days after enrollment. Table 2 shows the percentages, by gender, of patient satisfaction with services in the "very good" to "excellent" range.[1]

Respondents who rated the single item on overall satisfaction with services as being either "very good" or "excellent" were 65.4 percent of the total participant group (*n* = 251). Most males in the sample rated their overall service satisfaction as "very good" or "excellent" (70.8 percent). A smaller proportion of females in the sample rated their

TABLE 2. Patient Satisfaction Ratings of Respondents in Three Projects by Gender

	Percentage Among Males (n = 257)	Percentage Among Females (n = 127)
Services were "excellent" or "very good"	70.8%	54.3%
Staff answered questions "all" or "most times"	93.4%	93.0%
Patient was treated as an individual	96.5%	98.4%
Information received was easy to understand	95.3%	92.9%
Staff provided information about illness	92.2%	91.4%
Staff kept information private	98.4%	100.0%
Staff were available when needed	93.7%	95.2%
Services were available when needed	96.5%	93.1%
Patient would probably not go elsewhere for services	92.7%	92.9%

Note. Percentages represent patient satisfaction ratings of either "very good" or "excellent." The original response format for each satisfaction item was "fair/poor," "good," "very good," and "excellent."

overall service satisfaction as "very good" or "excellent" (54.3 percent).

Considering the individual satisfaction with services indicators, ratings for both male and female HIV/AIDS patients in each category considering services to be "very good" to "excellent" exceeded 90.0 percent. Research by Katz et al. (1997) noted that similar disparities between overall service satisfaction ratings and individual satisfaction indicators existed in their study samples. These disparities may be attributed to the fact that individual indicators focus on patient and provider interactions and treatment outcomes, while the overall satisfaction ratings reflect both provider relationships and perceptions about the administrative aspects of managed care. In other words, patients often express their satisfaction with services received from providers in the individual items and express their feelings about managed care, in general, in the overall satisfaction rating.

Procedure

As part of the cross-cutting evaluation, individual projects administered Modules 1 (Demographics-Contact Form) and 11 (Patient Satisfaction). In general, Module 1 was administered as part of the patient enrollment procedure; Module 11 was typically administered at regular intervals throughout the service episode. Staff representatives from each project site–usually program staff, rather than dedicated data collection staff–received training on the standardized use of these modules at three national steering committee meetings a year for the Cooperative Agreement. Repeated trainings were conducted to account for staff turnover over the course of the project and to prevent "drift" among continuing project staff. The national evaluators were available at all times to answer questions about administration when questions arose, and written instructions for administration were also provided.

Analysis Method

The modeling method used with these satisfaction ratings is called Exhaustive CHAID (Chi-squared Automatic Interaction Detector) (Biggs, de Ville, & Suen, 1991; Huba, 2000; Huba, Panter, & Melchior, 2000). CHAID is a method for analyzing outcomes that may be categorical (e.g., the single-item satisfaction with services index) or continuous (e.g., the patient satisfaction score obtained from the sum of the nine individual satisfaction indicators). Predictors may also be categorical or quantitative. Using a systematic checking algorithm, CHAID examines different combinations of the predictors to identify homogeneous groups of individuals who may be differentiated on the basis of the outcome measure. Hierarchical relationships may be determined empirically (using the optimization algorithm based on specified statistical significance levels), through theoretical choices, or both. The sample is split in a way to form a decision tree, which in general eases interpretability. The method and its interpretation are illustrated using two CHAID models for each major patient satisfaction outcome (the four-point global patient satisfaction index and the mean of the individual satisfaction items).

In the modeling analyses, the parent node was set at 10 and the child node was set at 5, except in situations where a missing value category was split for theoretical purposes. The alpha level of the statistical tests was set at .05, corrected for the number of statistical tests within a predictor using the Bonferroni method. All models were estimated using AnswerTree 2.0. The analyses for this paper were planned and conducted between 1998-2000 by Huba, Melchior, and Panter (1998-2000) for the Knowledge Base on HIV/AIDS Care available at *www.The MeasurementGroup.com/KB.htm.*

RESULTS

Effects of Need-Vulnerability Indicators and Gender on Patient Satisfaction (Single Item)

Table 3 shows the individual effects of the need-vulnerability-demographic predictors on program satisfaction levels using the final overall patient satisfaction rating. Of the 17 possible predictors, 14 significantly differentiated responses on the overall patient satisfaction rating. The significant predictors of satisfaction were: ethnicity, primary language, childcare needs, employment status, insurance coverage, alcohol problem, heroin use, crack use, other illicit drug use, criminal justice system involvement, sex work, sex with an injection drug user, sexual orientation, and gender. The percentage and number of patients falling into each response category based on the set of 17 predictors are shown in Table 3.

Model 1 for Patient Satisfaction with Services

The first CHAID model, the first three levels of which are shown in Figure 1, uses the dependent measure of the final overall patient satisfaction rating.[2] The predictor variables in the model were the 17 need-vulnerability-demographic indicators. Figure 1 is read in the following way: starting at the left side of the tree, if we consider all 384 individuals, a majority of patients rated their satisfaction with services received as being "very good" or "excellent" (65.4 percent). Because this model is entirely empirical–that is, it is fit to the data using purely mathematical rules–we can see in the second row of the tree (from the top) what the "best" way is to split the entire sample to differentiate those with the highest and lowest scores. It should be understood that only statistically significant groupings result from this analysis. As a consequence of this empirical rule, groups not shown should be interpreted as having comparable levels of satisfaction to that of the entire sample. As shown in Figure 1, the optimal split for the sample is based on race-ethnicity. Hispanic/Latino patients had relatively higher satisfaction in this model, whereas African American/Black patients had relatively lower levels. The satisfaction levels of African American/Black and Caucasian patients were further differentiated in terms of criminal justice system (CJS) involvement. In general, HIV/AIDS patients with no CJS involvement had greater satisfaction with care than

TABLE 3. Effects of Need-Vulnerability Factors on Patient Satisfaction Levels

Indicator	Fair/Poor % (n)	Good % (n)	Very Good % (n)	Excellent % (n)	χ^2	df
Age					0.87	1
Age 21-55	5.9 (22)	28.9 (108)	31.8 (119)	33.4 (125)		
Age > 55	10.0 (1)	20.0 (2)	10.0 (1)	60.0 (6)		
Race-Ethnicity					80.65***	3
African American/Black	7.6 (17)	39.6 (89)	36.0 (81)	16.9 (38)		
Hispanic/Latino	0.0 (0)	8.6 (5)	20.7 (12)	70.7 (41)		
Caucasian	6.1 (6)	16.3 (16)	27.6 (27)	50.0 (49)		
Combined Small Groups	0.0 (0)	0.0 (0)	0.0 (0)	100.0 (3)		
Primary Language					33.67***	1
English	6.8 (23)	31.8 (107)	32.1 (108)	29.4 (99)		
Not English	0.0 (0)	6.4 (3)	25.5 (12)	68.1 (32)		
Childcare needs					10.31*	3
No Childcare Needs	6.8 (21)	28.7 (88)	32.6 (100.0)	31.9 (98)		
1 Child Needs Care	0.0 (0)	37.5 (9)	29.2 (7)	33.3 (8)		
> 1 Child Needs Care	4.8 (1)	42.9 (9)	23.8 (5)	28.6 (6)		
Missing	3.1 (1)	12.5 (4)	25.0 (8)	59.4 (19)		
Highest Grade Completed					4.32	3
No HS (< 10)	7.7 (5)	32.3 (21)	32.3 (21)	27.7 (18)		
Some HS (10-11)	4.4 (4)	33.3 (30)	31.1 (28)	31.1 (28)		
HS Grad (12+)	6.0 (12)	26.5 (53)	33.0 (66.0)	34.5 (69)		
Missing	6.9 (2)	20.7 (6)	17.2 (5)	55.2 (16)		
Employment Status					14.54**	3
Employed	0.0 (0)	18.5 (5)	11.1 (3)	70.4 (19)		
Unemployed	2.0 (1)	32.7 (16)	26.5 (13)	38.8 (19)		
Disabled	6.6 (18)	29.9 (81)	34.7 (94)	28.8 (78)		
Missing	10.8 (4)	21.6 (8)	27.0 (10)	40.5 (15)		
Insurance Coverage					9.13*	3
Public Insurance	5.6 (19)	30.6 (103)	32.1 (108)	31.8 (107)		
Private Insurance	0.0 (0)	33.3 (2)	0.0 (0)	66.7 (4)		
No Insurance	0.0 (0)	0.0 (0)	0.0 (0)	100.0 (3)		
Missing	10.5 (4)	13.2 (5)	31.6 (12)	44.7 (17)		
Alcohol Problem					15.84**	3
No Alcohol Problem	5.6 (10)	33.3 (60)	36.1 (65)	25.0 (45)		
Prior Alcohol Problem	6.0 (6)	31.0 (31)	32.0 (32)	31.0 (31)		
Current Alcohol Problem	4.8 (1)	38.1 (8)	14.3 (3)	42.9 (9)		
Missing	7.2 (6)	13.3 (11)	24.1 (20)	55.4 (46)		
Heroin Use					36.93***	3
No Heroin	6.2 (11)	25.3 (45)	29.2 (52)	39.3 (70)		
Prior Heroin	5.5 (6)	44.0 (48)	39.5 (43)	11.0 (12)		
Current Heroin	0.0 (0)	60.0 (6)	40.0 (4)	0.0 (0)		
Missing	6.9 (6)	12.6 (11)	24.1 (21)	56.3 (49)		
Crack Use					36.68***	3
No Crack	2.9 (6)	28.4 (58)	35.8 (73)	32.8 (67)		
Prior Crack	10.3 (9)	43.7 (38)	29.9 (26)	16.1 (14)		
Current Crack	40.0 (2)	40.0 (2)	0.0 (0)	20.0 (1)		
Missing	6.8 (6)	13.6 (12)	23.9 (21)	55.7 (49)		
Other Illicit Drug Use					34.45***	3
No Other Drug	4.8 (6)	22.2 (28)	34.1 (43)	38.9 (49)		
Prior Other Drug	6.6 (9)	43.1 (59)	34.3 (47)	16.1 (22)		
Current Other Drug	5.7 (2)	34.3 (12)	25.7 (9)	34.3 (12)		
Missing	7.0 (6)	12.8 (11)	24.4 (21)	55.8 (48)		

TABLE 3 (continued)

Indicator	Fair/Poor % (n)	Good % (n)	Very Good % (n)	Excellent % (n)	χ^2	df
Criminal Justice System (CJS) Involvement					55.20***	3
No CJS Involvement	2.5 (4)	28.8 (47)	28.2 (46)	40.5 (66)		
Prior CJS Involvement	10.7 (13)	42.2 (51)	38.8 (47)	8.3 (10)		
Current CJS Involvement	0.0 (0)	20.0 (1)	20.0 (1)	60.0 (3)		
Missing	6.32 (6)	11.6 (11)	27.4 (26)	54.7 (52)		
Sex Work					27.34***	3
No Sex Work	5.7 (14)	31.6 (78)	34.0 (84)	28.7 (71)		
Prior Sex Work	7.1 (3)	45.2 (19)	33.3 (14)	14.3 (6)		
Current Sex Work	0.0 (0)	100.0 (1)	0.0 (0)	0.0 (0)		
Missing	6.4 (6)	12.8 (12)	23.4 (22)	57.5 (54)		
Sex with Injection Drug User (IDU)					16.09**	3
No Sex with IDU	0.9 (1)	24.3 (27)	36.0 (40)	38.7 (43)		
Prior Sex with IDU	10.4 (8)	40.3 (31)	28.6 (22)	20.8 (16)		
Current Sex with IDU	0.0 (0)	50.0 (4)	37.5 (3)	12.5 (1)		
Missing	7.5 (14)	25.5 (48)	29.3 (55)	37.8 (71)		
Housing Status					6.25	3
Own Home	5.0 (10)	30.5 (61)	25.5 (51)	39.0 (78)		
Friend's Home	7.1 (9)	30.7 (39)	39.4 (50)	22.8 (29)		
Unstable Housing	0.0 (0)	26.1 (6)	43.5 (10)	30.4 (7)		
Missing	11.8 (4)	11.8 (4)	26.5 (9)	50.0 (17)		
Sexual Orientation					27.38***	3
Gay/Lesbian	4.9 (5)	9.8 (10)	33.3 (34)	52.0 (53)		
Bisexual	11.5 (3)	23.1 (6)	26.9 (7)	38.5 (10)		
Heterosexual	6.5 (15)	35.9 (83)	32.5 (75)	25.1 (58)		
Unknown	0.0 (0)	44.0 (11)	16.0 (4)	40.0 (10)		
Gender					8.32**	1
Male	5.8 (15)	23.4 (60)	32.7 (84)	38.1 (98)		
Female	6.3 (8)	39.4 (50)	28.4 (36)	26.0 (33)		

*$p < .05$, **$p < .01$, ***$p < .001$
Note. "Prior" denotes the behavior occurred prior to the past 30 days; "Current" denotes the behavior occurred within the past 30 days. The chi-square values shown here are for the relationship of a nominal variable to an ordinal variable (in this case, the overall quality rating) and were calculated using Goodman's (1979) formula in the AnswerTree program, version 2.1 (SPSS, 1999).

did those with prior or current CJS involvement. Note, however, that there were very few individuals in this sample with current (past 30 days) CJS involvement reported. Further differences in the sample based on satisfaction levels diverged from this point in the model. Among African American/Black patients with missing data as to CJS involvement, those with public insurance reported greater satisfaction than did those with missing data as to insurance coverage. Finally, of those in this group with public insurance, the small sub-sample was split by gender. On the other side of the model, Caucasian HIV/AIDS patients with no CJS involvement were split by gender, with a small group of females having lower satisfaction levels than males.

FIGURE 1. First Two Splits in a Fully Empirical Model of a Single-Item Patient Satisfaction Rating and Need-Vulnerability-Demographic Factors

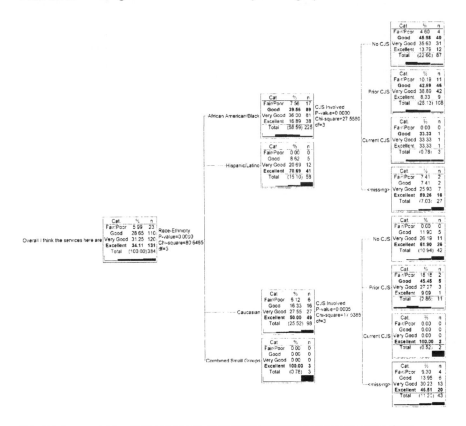

Note. This is a completely empirical model with only statistically significant homogenous groups shown.

Model 2 for Patient Satisfaction with Services (Gender-Specific)

In building the tree models, it is possible to split the sample in a way the user specifies, usually on the basis of theory or prevailing wisdom in a "forced" way, and to combine various forced steps with ones that are purely empirical or optimally guided by the data. Figure 2 shows the first two splits in a model in which the first split was forced to be gender. Of the 257 male HIV/AIDS patients, 70.8 percent rated the services they received as being "very good" or "excellent," compared to 54.3 percent of the 127 female HIV/AIDS patients who rated the services they received as being "very good" or "excellent" at the

FIGURE 2. First Two Splits in a Model of a Single-Item Patient Satisfaction Rating and Need-Vulnerability-Demographic Factors: Gender at First Split with Subsequent Fully Empirical Model

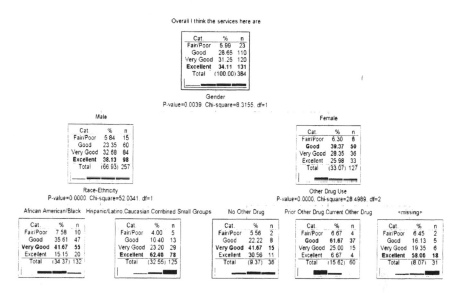

Note. This model was empirically derived after the first split by gender. Only statistically significant groupings are included in the model.

most recent assessment. Next, for males and females separately, we examined a model based on empirical criteria to obtain the best fit to the observed data. Satisfaction levels among males are differentiated based on ethnicity and CJS involvement. Satisfaction levels among females are differentiated based on illicit drug use, ethnicity, and sex work. Among the HIV/AIDS patients, African Americans had lower reported levels of satisfaction. Regardless of racial-ethnic background, the next factor to predict patient satisfaction levels was CJS involvement. Although they are shown as separate categories in the model, note that the number of males with current (past 30 days) CJS involvement is quite small. Satisfaction with care among female HIV/AIDS patients was first split by drug use, with those having no use of drugs other than crack or heroin reporting relatively higher levels of satisfaction.

Most female HIV/AIDS patients in the sample with either prior or current drug abuse reported their satisfaction with services as "good"

(61.7 percent). The females with no history of illicit drug use (other than crack cocaine or heroin) were further divided by race-ethnicity, although the size of these groups becomes quite small. Finally, African American female patients with no other illicit drug use are further split by involvement in sex work, although the prior sex work and missing data groups each include fewer than five individuals.

Effects of Need-Vulnerability Indicators and Gender on Total Patient Satisfaction Scores

As an alternative to using the overall satisfaction item response as the dependent measure, we also examined the relationship of need-vulnerability-demographic indicators to the total satisfaction scores. Table 4 shows the individual effects of the 17 need-vulnerability-demographic indicators on patient satisfaction levels using the index based on the sum of the nine patient satisfaction items. Eleven of the 17 possible predictors significantly differentiated responses on the total satisfaction scores: race-ethnicity, primary language, highest grade completed, employment status, heroin use, crack use, other illicit drug use, criminal justice system involvement, sex work, sex with an IDU, and sexual orientation. Some effects were small. The mean and standard deviation for the total satisfaction score, as well as the number of persons in each group based on these 17 indicators, are shown in Table 4.

Model 1 for Total Patient Satisfaction with Program

Figure 3 shows the first two splits in a purely empirical model fit to the most recent total satisfaction score. Note that this figure looks slightly different than Figures 1 and 2 because the dependent variable of total satisfaction rating is now a quantitative (continuous) variable rather than a categorical one. In the entire sample ($N = 384$), the satisfaction score was 30.80 on a scale of 9 to 36, with 9 being "least satisfied" and 36 being "most satisfied." The small graph in the box shows the distribution of the total service satisfaction scores.

A tree was developed in which the patients were split using an entirely empirical set of rules so as to best fit the data overall (shown in Figure 3). The optimal way to split the sample initially was by race-ethnicity. African American/Black respondents had slightly lower total satisfaction scores than did other racial-ethnic groups. Among African American/Black and Caucasian groups, satisfaction scores were further

TABLE 4. Effects of Need-Vulnerability Factors on Total Satisfaction Score

Indicator	*M*	*SD*	*n*	%	*F*	*df*
Age					0.66	1, 382
Age 21-55	30.77	3.95	374	97.4		
Age > 55	31.80	3.65	10	2.6		
Race-Ethnicity					20.52***	3, 380
African American/Black	29.61	3.16	225	58.6		
Hispanic/Latino	33.26	3.38	58	15.1		
Caucasian	32.96	4.78	98	25.5		
Combined Small Groups	34.00	3.46	3	0.8		
Language not English					22.37***	1, 382
English	30.45	3.93	337	87.8		
Not English	33.29	3.08	47	12.2		
Childcare needs					2.47	3, 380
No Childcare Needs	30.71	3.97	307	80.0		
1 Child Needs Care	30.92	2.90	24	6.3		
> 1 Child Needs Care	29.57	4.44	21	5.5		
Missing	32.38	3.66	32	8.3		
Highest Grade Completed					3.07*	3, 380
No HS (< Grade 10)	30.22	3.88	65	16.9		
Some HS (Grade 10-11)	30.23	4.27	90	23.4		
HS grad (Grade 12+ or GED)	31.00	3.73	200	52.1		
Missing	32.48	4.01	29	7.6		
Employment Status					4.97**	3, 380
Employed	33.52	2.56	27	7.0		
Unemployed	31.00	3.88	49	12.8		
Disabled	30.52	3.84	271	70.6		
Missing	30.54	4.87	37	9.6		
Insurance Coverage					2.06	3, 380
Public Insurance	30.68	3.84	337	87.8		
Private Insurance	32.83	2.64	6	1.6		
No Insurance	35.33	0.58	3	0.8		
Missing	31.13	4.83	38	9.9		
Alcohol Problem					2.52	3, 380
No Alcohol Problem	30.89	3.48	180	46.9		
Prior Alcohol Problem	30.31	4.12	100	26.0		
Current Alcohol Problem	38.86	4.34	21	5.5		
Missing	31.81	4.43	83	21.6		
Heroin Use					9.48***	3, 380
No Heroin	31.28	3.77	178	46.4		
Prior Heroin	29.28	3.55	109	28.4		
Current Heroin	29.30	1.25	10	2.6		
Missing	31.87	4.37	87	22.7		
Crack Use					6.82***	3, 380
No Crack	31.01	3.46	204	53.1		
Prior Crack	29.36	4.14	87	22.7		
Current Crack	28.80	4.66	5	1.3		
Missing	31.83	4.37	88	22.9		
Other Illicit Drug Use					6.95***	3, 380
No Other Drug	31.35	3.70	126	32.8		
Prior Other Drug	29.72	3.53	137	35.7		
Current Other Drug	30.34	4.24	35	9.1		
Missing	31.90	4.38	86	22.4		

TABLE 4 (continued)

Indicator	M	SD	n	%	F	df
Criminal Justice System (CJS) Involved					11.81***	3, 380
No CJS Involvement	31.28	3.79	163	42.5		
Prior CJS Involvement	29.16	3.38	121	31.5		
Current CJS Involvement	32.20	3.56	5	1.3		
Missing	31.99	4.25	95	24.7		
Sex Work					4.64**	3, 380
No Sex Work	30.61	3.61	247	64.3		
Prior Sex Work	29.43	4.51	42	11.0		
Current Sex Work	29.00	--	1	0.3		
Missing	31.93	4.27	94	24.5		
Sex with Injection Drug User (IDU)					4.75**	3, 380
No Sex with IDU	31.63	3.83	111	28.9		
Prior Sex with IDU	29.53	3.80	77	20.1		
Current Sex with IDU	29.50	2.88	8	2.1		
Missing	30.88	3.98	188	49.0		
Housing Status					2.12	3, 380
Own Home	31.08	4.00	200	52.1		
Friend's Home	30.12	3.67	127	33.1		
Unstable Housing	31.78	2.98	23	6.0		
Missing	31.03	4.89	34	8.9		
Sexual Orientation					3.59*	3, 380
Gay/Lesbian	31.83	4.46	102	26.6		
Bisexual	30.04	5.27	26	6.8		
Heterosexual	30.39	3.47	231	60.2		
Unknown	31.08	3.62	25	6.5		
Gender					1.76	1, 382
Male	31.98	4.10	257	66.9		
Female	30.42	3.60	127	33.1		

Note. *$p < .05$, **$p < .01$, ***$p < .001$; "Prior" denotes the behavior occurred prior to the past 30 days; "Current" denotes the behavior occurred within the past 30 days.

predicted by CJS involvement. Patients with prior CJS involvement had lower satisfaction scores than other groups based on CJS status. In addition, African American patients with unknown CJS involvement were further split by insurance status. Finally, among Caucasian patients with no CJS involvement, there was a gender difference, with males reporting greater satisfaction with care than did females.

Model 2 for Total Patient Satisfaction with Program (Gender-Specific)

As an alternative to the model shown in Figure 3 for total patient satisfaction scores, we also developed a model for the same data in which the split at the first level was specified to be gender. Then, within each gender, we allowed the data to be split empirically into the

FIGURE 3. First Two Splits in a Fully Empirical Model of Total Patient Satisfaction Scores and Need-Vulnerability-Demographic Factors

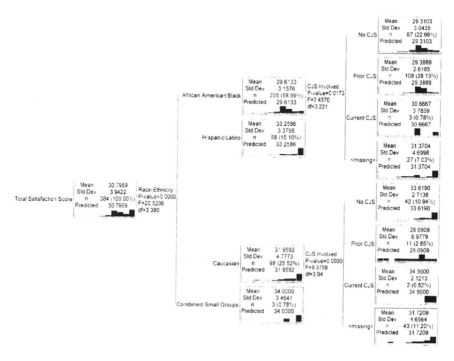

Note. This empirical model is based on the mean of the total score for nine satisfaction items. Total scores were determined by summing patient rankings for each of the nine items. Each item could be ranked from 1–least satisfied, to 4–most satisfied.

groups that produced the greatest differences. The first two splits in this model are given in Figure 4. For male HIV/AIDS patients, the patterns of total satisfaction scores are significantly related to race-ethnicity and CJS involvement. The pattern of results for males is quite similar to that shown in the previous model (Figure 3). Among female HIV/AIDS patients, the sample is best differentiated by race-ethnicity, employment status, and highest grade completed. In this sample, African American female patients had lower satisfaction scores than did Hispanic/Latina or Caucasian female patients. Among the African American females, those who were employed had higher satisfaction scores than others. African American/Black females who were unemployed or disabled were further split by education level, with those with less than a tenth grade education having the lowest satisfaction scores.

FIGURE 4. First Two Splits in a Model of Patient Satisfaction Scores and Need-Vulnerability-Demographic Factors: Gender at First Split with Subsequent Fully Empirical Model

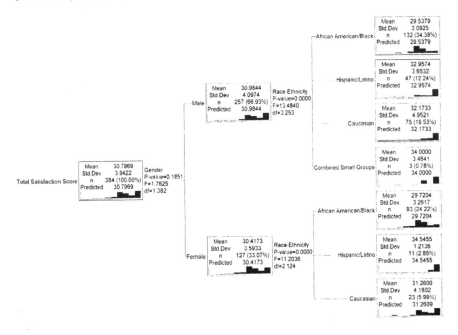

Note. The gender split in this model was forced. All subsequent groupings were derived empirically. The mean score is based on the sum of patients' ratings on nine satisfaction with service items.

DISCUSSION

Findings from the three demonstration projects indicate that males were more satisfied overall with these managed care models than were females. While this finding holds for the single item rating of patient satisfaction, this was not the case for the results involving the summed patient satisfaction score. In this sample, over 90 percent of both males and females rated individual items of service satisfaction as "very good" to "excellent." The gender difference in the overall satisfaction rating is consistent with reports in the literature, where men tend to rate satisfaction with managed care programs higher than do women (e.g., Katz et al., 1997). Current HIV medical care systems often do not meet the needs of women, especially for African American women (e.g., Eversley, Israelski, Smith, & Kunwar, 1998), which may in part explain the obtained difference in reported satisfaction levels.

As noted earlier, the phenomenon of lower ratings on overall satisfaction with services compared to higher ratings on individual satisfaction items has been obtained in previous studies of managed care with Medicaid populations. HIV-infected individuals tend to report satisfaction with most specific aspects of their medical care (e.g., patient provider interaction-interpersonal relationships and communications)–higher than they rate satisfaction in general. This difference often indicates satisfaction with particular providers rather than the system of care (Katz et al., 1997; Wilson et al., 1998). It is important for states to consider these rating differences and measurement consequences as they move HIV/AIDS populations and Medicaid populations into managed care. The potential wholesale movement of populations into managed care can result in considerable dissatisfaction with services, regardless of extremely high ratings of patient satisfaction with their healthcare providers. Overall dissatisfaction with the managed care system by patients may have a profound negative impact on their adherence to treatment.

Given the complicated dynamics surrounding the movement of HIV/AIDS patients into managed care, the three providers discussed here did an excellent job of building integrated systems of care and paying continuous attention to the full spectrum of patient needs. It is clear from the strong results on patient-provider interactions that most participants rated services extremely highly. African American women were relatively less satisfied with these services than any other sample cohort. This group has historically experienced significant barriers to accessing care. In part, their lower overall satisfaction with service ratings may be a product of both historic issues and a current sense of helplessness at being "forced" by states to enroll in a managed care environment. Even in this group, however, their mean score for satisfaction with services fell within ranking services as "good" to "very good."

Providers who enter the managed care area need to be sensitive to both the physiological needs and the cultural issues of the special populations they serve. Providing treatment for HIV/AIDS patients who require intensive care can force providers to manage costs instead of care. The providers in this study developed appropriate cost-efficient rates for care, while providing effective, community-based service delivery models.

AUTHOR NOTES

This study was supported in part by Health Resources and Services Administration (HRSA), HIV/AIDS Bureau (HAB), Special Projects of National Significance (SPNS) Grant Number 5 U90 HA 00030-05 for the work of the Evaluation and Dissemination Center and by grants to the individual projects. This article's contents are solely the responsibility of the authors and do not necessarily represent the official view of the funding agency. From University of Washington, School of Social Work & The Measurement Group (D. Cherin), from The Measurement Group (G. Huba, L. Melchior), from the East Boston Neighborhood Health Center (J. Steinberg), from AIDS Healthcare Foundation (P. Reis), and from the Health Resources and Services Administration (K. Marconi). The analyses for this paper were planned and conducted between 1998-2000 by Huba, Melchior, and Panter (1998-2000) for the Knowledge Base on HIV/AIDS Care available at *www.TheMeasurementGroup. com/KB.htm*. Special thanks to Rupinder K. Sidhu, Cindy T. Le, Chermeen Elavia, and Kimberly Ishihara for help with manuscript preparation, to Jocelyn Medina and Katherine Ellingson for help with data processing, and to the late Diana E. Brief, PhD, for help with data management, all of The Measurement Group.

NOTES

1. Human Subjects Protection Committees at each site determined if informed consent for participation in the evaluation was required, or if the data were collected as part of the usual quality improvement process, and hence exempt. All data collection at all sites was voluntary for clients and providers and, hence, these data do have certain non-random patterns of missing observations.

2. Because of space limitations due to printing at this size, the models shown in Figures 1 through 4 are limited to three levels (two splits) each. Supplemental figures showing the complete models in full color are available online at *www.TheMeasurement Group.com/HHC/mcsatis.htm*.

REFERENCES

Biggs, D., de Ville, B., & Suen, E. (1991). A method of choosing multiway partitions for classification and decision trees. *Journal of Applied Statistics, 18*, 49-62.

Eversley, R., Israelski, D., Smith, S., & Kunwar, P. (1998). Satisfaction with medical care is associated with race, HIV symptoms and recovery from substance abuse among HIV-infected women. *International Conference on AIDS, 12*, 815-816. (Abstract No. 42214).

Huba, G. J. (2001). Introduction: Evaluating HIV/AIDS Treatment Programs for Underserved and Vulnerable Patients, Innovative Methods and Findings. *Home Health Care Services Quarterly: The Journal of Community Care, 19*(1/2), 1-6.

Huba, G. J., Melchior, L. A., De Veauuse, N., Hillary, K., Singer, B., & Marconi, K. (1998). A national program of AIDS capitated care projects and their evaluation. *Home Health Care Services Quarterly, 17* (1), 3-30.

Huba, G. J., Melchior, L. A., Panter, A. T., Brown, V. B., & Larson, T. L. (2000). A national program of AIDS care projects and their cross-cutting evaluation: The HRSA SPNS Cooperative Agreements. *Drugs & Society, 16*(1/2), 5-29.

Huba, G. J., Melchior, L. A., Panter, A. T., Smereck, G., Meredith, K., Cherin, D. A., Richardson-Nassif, K., German, V. F., Rohweder, C., Brown, V. B., McDonald, S., Kaplan, J., Stanton, A., Chase, P., Jean-Louis, E., Gallagher, T., Steinberg, J., Reis, P., Mundy, L., & Larson, T. A. (2000). Psychometric scaling of a disenfranchisement index for HIV service need. Manuscript in preparation.

Huba, G. J., Melchior, L. A., & Panter, A. T. (1998-2000). Knowledge Base on HIV/ AIDS Care. Online: *www.TheMeasurementGroup.com/KB.htm.*

Huba, G. J., Melchior, L. A., Staff of The Measurement Group, & the HRSA SPNS Cooperative Agreement Projects. (1997a). *Module 1: Demographics-Contact Form.* Online: *www.TheMeasurementGroup.com/modules.htm.*

Huba, G. J., Melchior, L. A., Staff of The Measurement Group, & the HRSA SPNS Cooperative Agreement Projects. (1997b). *Module 11: Patient Satisfaction Survey.* Online: *www.TheMeasurementGroup.com/modules.htm.*

Huba, G. J., Panter, A. T., & Melchior, L. A. (2000). Empirical modeling of patient characteristics and services using sample partitioning, interaction detection, or classification tree methods: Practical issues and recommendations. Manuscript in preparation.

Jatulis, D. E., Bundek, N. I., & Legorreta, A. P. (1997). Identifying predictors of satisfaction with access to medical care and quality of care. *American Journal of Medical Quality, 12* (1), 11-18.

Katz, M. H., Marx, R., Douglas, J. M., Bolan, G. A., Park, M., Gurley, R., & Buchbinder, S. P. (1997). Insurance type and satisfaction with medical care among HIV-infected men. *Journal of Acquired Immune Deficiency Syndrome, 14* (1), 35-43.

Kitahata, M. M., Holmes, K. K., Wagner, E. H., & Gooding, T. D. (1998). Caring for persons with HIV infection in a managed care environment. *The American Journal of Medicine, 104* (6), 511-515.

Powell, A., O'Neill, J. F., Holloway, J. E., & Gomez, M. G. (1998). US Federal strategies for increasing involvement by people living with HIV (PLWH) in planning for HIV services. *International Conference on AIDS, 12*, 104. (Abstract No. 12453).

SPSS (1999). *AnswerTree*, version 2.1 (computer software).

Weiss, B. D., & Senf, J. H. (1990). Patient satisfaction survey instrument for use in health maintenance organization. *Medical Care, 28* (5), 434-445.

Wilson, I. B., Sullivan, L. M., & Weissman, J. S. (1998). Costs and outcomes of AIDS care: Comparing a health maintenance organization with fee-for-service systems in the Boston Health Study. *Journal of Acquired Immune Deficiency Syndrome, 17* (5), 424-432.

Index

AIDS. *See* HIV/AIDS
AIDS Healthcare Foundation, 10,22,
　107,108
Aranda-Naranjo, Barbara, 5

Barriers. *See* Service barriers
Brown, Vivian B., 5,7-27,29-51,53-75,
　77-102

Care services. *See* HIV/AIDS services
Center for Community Health
　Education and Research
　(CCHER) Haitian
　Community AIDS Outreach
　Project, 10,21,33,57,82
CHAID (Chi-squared Automatic
　Interaction Detector), 3-4,
　15-16,39-40,112
Chase, Paul, 7-27
Cherin, David A., 5,7-27,77-102,
　103-125
Client satisfaction, 78-79,97-99. *See*
　also Patient satisfaction
　indicators for, 84-86
　Module 11 Survey, 84,85-86
　research design for, 81-87
　research results for, 88-97
　service delivery and, 79-80
Cocaine users. *See* Crack-cocaine
　users
Community-Based Organizations
　(CBOs), 2-3
　client satisfaction and, 78-80
Cooperative Agreement Projects. *See*
　SPNS Cooperative
　Agreement Projects
Crack-cocaine users

need-vulnerability scores of, 16-20
unmet needs of, 47
Cultural sensitivity, 31-32

Designs, research. *See* Research
　designs
Drug abuse. *See* Substance abuse

East Boston Neighborhood Health
　Center, 10,22,107,108
End of life care, 22
Exhaustive CHAID method. *See*
　CHAID (Chi-squared
　Automatic Interaction
　Detector)

The Fortune Society, 10,22,33,57,82

Gallagher, Tracey, 7-27,29-51,53-75,
　77-102
Gender
　need-vulnerability index and, 23
　patient satisfaction and, 116-118
German, Victor F., 7-27,29-51,53-75
Grace, William, 5
Group Health Association of America
　(GHAA), 105

Healthcare providers, 55-56
HIV/AIDS
　changing populations impacted by,
　　8-9
　epidemiological trends, 30
　projects studying populations of,
　　9-13

　　　127

Printed and bound by CPI Group (UK) Ltd, Croydon, CR0 4YY

17/10/2024

01775686-0009